The Real Food Athlete

Nutrition for performance, recovery, fat adaptation and athletic longevity

Steph Lowe

All rights reserved. No part of this book may be reproduced in part or in its entirety, in any form or by any electronic or mechanical means including information storage and retrieval systems, unless written permission by the author has first been obtained.

Published in 2016 by Steph Lowe
www.thenaturalnutritionist.com.au

© The Natural Nutritionist 2016

Catalogue-In-Publication details available from the National Library of Australia

ISBN: 978-0-646-95709-8 (pbk)

Photography by Sarah Craven Photography
Graphic Design by Ripe Designs

Book layout and design
by Publicious Pty Ltd
www.publicious.com.au

Published with the assistance of
Publicious Pty Ltd

This book contains the personal opinions of the author and is not designed to treat all health conditions. Please consult your health care practitioner if you are unsure.

The author disclaims any liability or responsibility for any loss or damage incurred directly or indirectly as a result of the information contained in this book.

To my nephews Hudson and Parker – believe in
your dreams and create a life that you love.

Foreword

The Real Food Athlete is a balanced, useful and practical approach that can help athletes of all levels achieve better endurance performance and health.

In particular, the book takes the guesswork out of becoming more fat adapted, not only in providing valuable information, but with one of the key components to make it all happen — recipes.

The many recipes are healthy, practical and easy to prepare — and yes, really made from real food. The accompanying food photos are worth a thousand mouth-watering words.

The book's important message is clear. Sticking to real food not only improves your health, speeds recovery, and helps you burn more body fat for increased energy and getting leaner, it can also help you continue on your health and fitness quest well into the future.

This fantastic book serves as an excellent guide that athletes from beginner to elite can review regularly to help guide them toward optimal human potential.

In a world full of fake food and fake nutritional guidance, this is a refreshingly real book is by the real Steph, and I hope you enjoy it as much as I have in the endeavour to help everyone become a *Real Food Athlete*.

– Dr. Philip Maffetone
Author, *The Big Book of Endurance Training and Racing*

Our Real Food Athletes

"I have been working with Steph at The Natural Nutritionist for over a year now. As a triathlete, nutrition is incredibly important. My day to day nutrition and race day fuelling are now based on real food. It hasn't only helped my health but it has had a massive impact on my recovery and my immune system. My body is more in balance now. Being healthy and recovering well has had a massive impact on my training consistency and "consistency = performance". I have enjoyed PBs in the last year at the 5km, half-marathon and sprint triathlon distance and am excited where I can take this in 2016 with my long course triathlon goals."

– David. P

"As I have always been interested in health and wellbeing I knew that eating a variety of whole foods is so important to perform at your best. I started CrossFit 2 years ago and needed a little extra guidance as my body demanded more intake and I wasn't recovering as well as I'd liked. I met with Steph at The Natural Nutritionist and she gave me some great advice and taught me what feels best, which foods aid my workouts, and most importantly, at what times. Now I recover really well, my performance is always improving and I have never felt healthier."

– Kylie. W

"After an extensive break from the sport I returned to triathlon shortly after turning 40. I was fat, lazy, unmotivated and just had the proverbial "mid-life crisis". Well how the sport had changed! All the gels, power bars and energy drinks obviously meant racing nutrition was now so easy. Well after 18 gels, 6 energy bars and countless high sugar drinks at Ironman Port Macquarie, in 2013, my stomach and body was screaming at me "there must be a better way". So I embarked on my search for the low carb/high fat alternative, The Paleo Way, and there was a plethora of information to be found. So I took a bit of this, a bit of that and once again I thought I had this all sorted. So I line up at Ironman Busselton, in 2014, good swim, solid bike and was feeling fantastic. Then 30 minutes into the marathon the 'bonk' came from nowhere, the earth opened up, swallowed me hole, and spat me back out as I crossed the finish line! Then after 5 hours in the medical tent I again knew: "I absolutely needed to find a better way!"

So as I once again embarked on my new quest for answers, I'm pleased to say that I found Steph Lowe, from The Natural Nutritionist. Since then I have absolutely not looked back. Over the past 12 months Steph has mentored me, guided me and most importantly has shown me the benefits of just eating real food. I've learnt how simple it is to plan meals, to eat the right foods at the right times and race fuelling strategies! My energy levels have become stable, recovery is so much faster, which obviously aids in improved training sessions, and I now have my health back. Losing 28 kilograms in the process whilst eating bacon might also be an added bonus. Thanks Steph, Just Eating Real Food has turned my life around!

– Scott. G

"Around 12 months ago I went in search of someone that could assist me in not only improving my athletic performance as an endurance athlete, but who could also support me to make some much needed changes to my nutrition to ease the multitude of GI issues and hormonal imbalances I was experiencing, and to help me change my mindset on what was 'healthy'. I've always invested in my health and fitness, but I needed some support to take it to the next level.

With Steph's support and guidance, 12 months on, my life has changed. I no longer have daily GI issues, I have more energy, I have a far better relationship with food, I'm well on the way to correcting my hormonal imbalances and I'm enjoying creating and eating amazing, delicious, nutrient dense foods. Whilst these changes may seem small and gradual at the time, they've had a huge impact on my life; from an athletic point of view this looks like a 9min marathon PB and completing my first ultra marathon with no GI issues (Freedom Fuel is my saviour!) and more broadly I'm a happier, healthier, more educated and more positive person than ever."

– Eliza. H

"Venturing into the world of long course triathlon and ultra distance running called for a renewed approach to the way I was eating. After scouring the internet for resources on how best to fuel my body during and after training, I came across Steph and all the awesome content she has on her website. It was through reading her blog and sending her a few cheeky emails, I was able to really turn my focus around and take my racing and life to next level performance. Initially, Steph and her ethos was the catalyst for a career change into nutrition and triathlon coaching. I owe a lot to the well researched, clearly conveyed information Steph has so kindly shared with everyone over the years. Congrats Steph… love your work."

– Scott. F

A note before we dive in

Before we get real...You want the facts, we all do, so let me direct you a set of key resources your should familiarise with in conjunction with The Real Food Athlete.

I have designed this book to be simple to understand and a resource to help you implement the strategies required to change your life. It is an accumulation of my work since starting The Natural Nutritionist in 2011. The experts to follow have done the research for us, so I have chosen not to repeat this in The Real Food Athlete. Please see below for further information and references:

1. *The Real Meal Revolution* by Professor Tim Noakes, Jonno Proudfoot and Sally-Ann Creed.
2. *Good Calories, Bad Calories* by Gary Taubes.
3. *It Starts With Food* by Dallas and Melissa Hartwig.
4. *The Big Book of Endurance Training and Racing* by Dr Philip Maffetone.
5. *The Art and Science of Low Carbohydrate Performance* by Jeff Volek and Stephen Phinney.
6. *Metabolic Efficiency Training* by Bob Seebohar.
7. *Primal Endurance* by Mark Sisson and Brad Kearns.

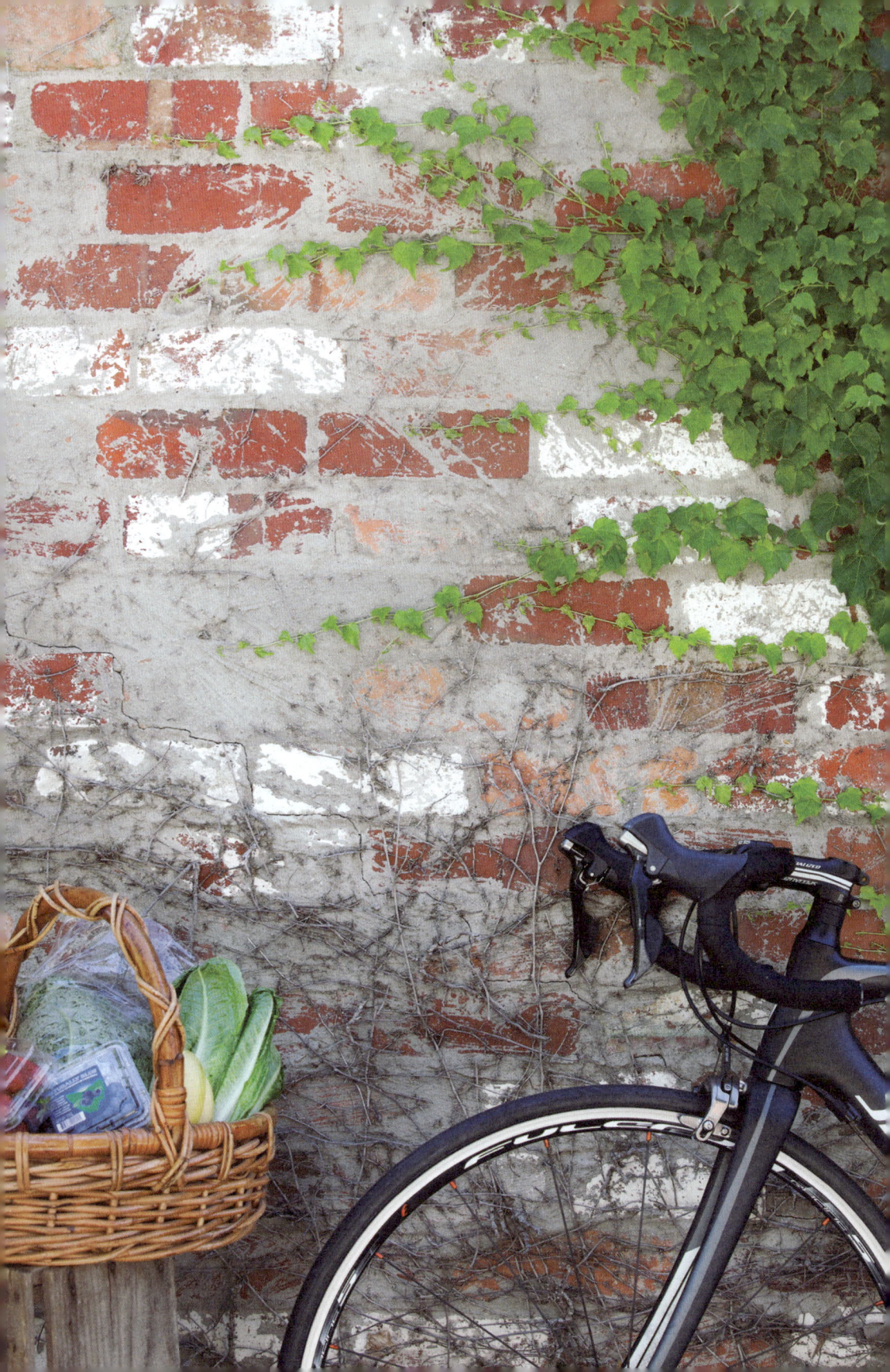

Contents

Introduction — 1
Welcome to the Real Food Athlete — 1
The Real Steph Lowe — 3

Part 1: The Technical Stuff — 5
The "foods" you need to quit — 6
Do I need to go Paleo? — 11
The importance of gut health — 13

Part 2: Becoming a Fat Adapted Athlete — 17
Fat adaptation 101 — 18
The benefits of fat adaptation — 20
Common mistakes to avoid — 28
Am I a fat burner? — 30
Your 12-week timeline — 32
What about strength athletes? — 34
What about yoga? — 36

Part 3: Just Eat Real Food (JERF) — 39
JERF — 40
How to build your plate — 41
Carbs, carbs, carbs! — 45
Kitchen makeover — 47
Gut health 101 — 68
Eating out — 72
Travelling — 74

Part 4: Recipes 77

Brekkie	79
Snack attack	107
Salad days	123
On the side	139
Quick and easy mains	153
Real good condiments	181
Sports nutrition power foods	191
Gut-loving eats	213

Welcome to the Real Food Athlete

I believe everyone is an athlete. Whether you're an eight-hour Ironman, or training for your first 5km, you ARE an athlete. Yogi? Athlete. CrossFitter? Athlete. I hope you see yourself that way and recognise the benefits of natural nutrition when it comes to living a healthy and high performance lifestyle.

Yes, we're talking **REAL food.** Food that comes out of the ground, off a tree or from an animal – I believe this will always be the most nutrient dense and whole food source of nutrition. If you're just starting out, the biggest change you can make to improve your health (and indeed your performance) is to significantly reduce or eliminate your packaged food consumption.

The Real Food Athlete was born because of the need to dispel the myths of sports nutrition companies and their multi-million dollar marketing campaigns, dogmatic carbohydrate guidelines and the recommendations that all athletes must fuel off 60-90 grams of carbohydrates per hour.

I'll teach you why you don't need Gatorade, commercial gels or the pasta party. You'll learn the benefits of real food, becoming a fat adapted athlete and how to fuel naturally in training and racing for optimal performance, recovery and athletic longevity.

Thousands of athletes worldwide are implementing these strategies, and now it's time for you to experience the benefits and become a Real Food Athlete. For those of you that already are, congratulations! This book will continue to inspire your real food journey and provide you with a resource you can share with your friends, family, fellow athletes and even your coach. The more we speak our language, the more we educate the world.

Let's do this together, team.

Steph x

P.S. Don't forget to share your success stories and kitchen creations on social media to keep our message spreading. @thenaturalnutritionist #thenaturalnutritionist #RFA #realfoodathlete #JERF

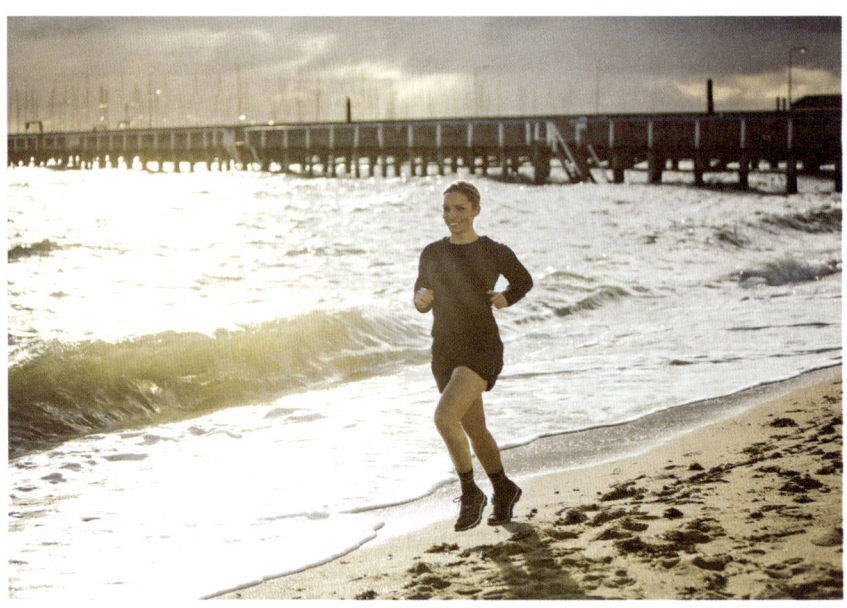

The Real Steph Lowe

As a Sports Nutritionist, triathlete and cashew butter addict from Melbourne, Victoria, it's safe to say, I know a bit about eating for optimal performance. My company The Natural Nutritionist, specialises in real food education, high performance fat loss, and metabolic efficiency for athletes.

A little more about me:
- I'm a long course triathlete currently taking a break from racing to reset the body and mind.
- I have personally been gluten free over ten years now, simply because it makes me happy. You can read more about my story online at www.thenaturalnutritionist.com.au/my-story-finally.
- I have an undergraduate degree in Sport and Exercise Science (James Cook University, Townsville).
- I have a postgraduate degree in Human Nutrition (Deakin University, Melbourne) and am one subject away from completing my masters.
- I promise you it's easier than you think. Only a few years ago all I could "cook" was a tuna salad. Seriously. So dive in, and in no time you will be sans recipe.
- How did I get to where I am now? Passion and consistency. My biggest piece of advice is to dive straight in – study, blog, create, share and enjoy the journey. Do what you love, love what you do!

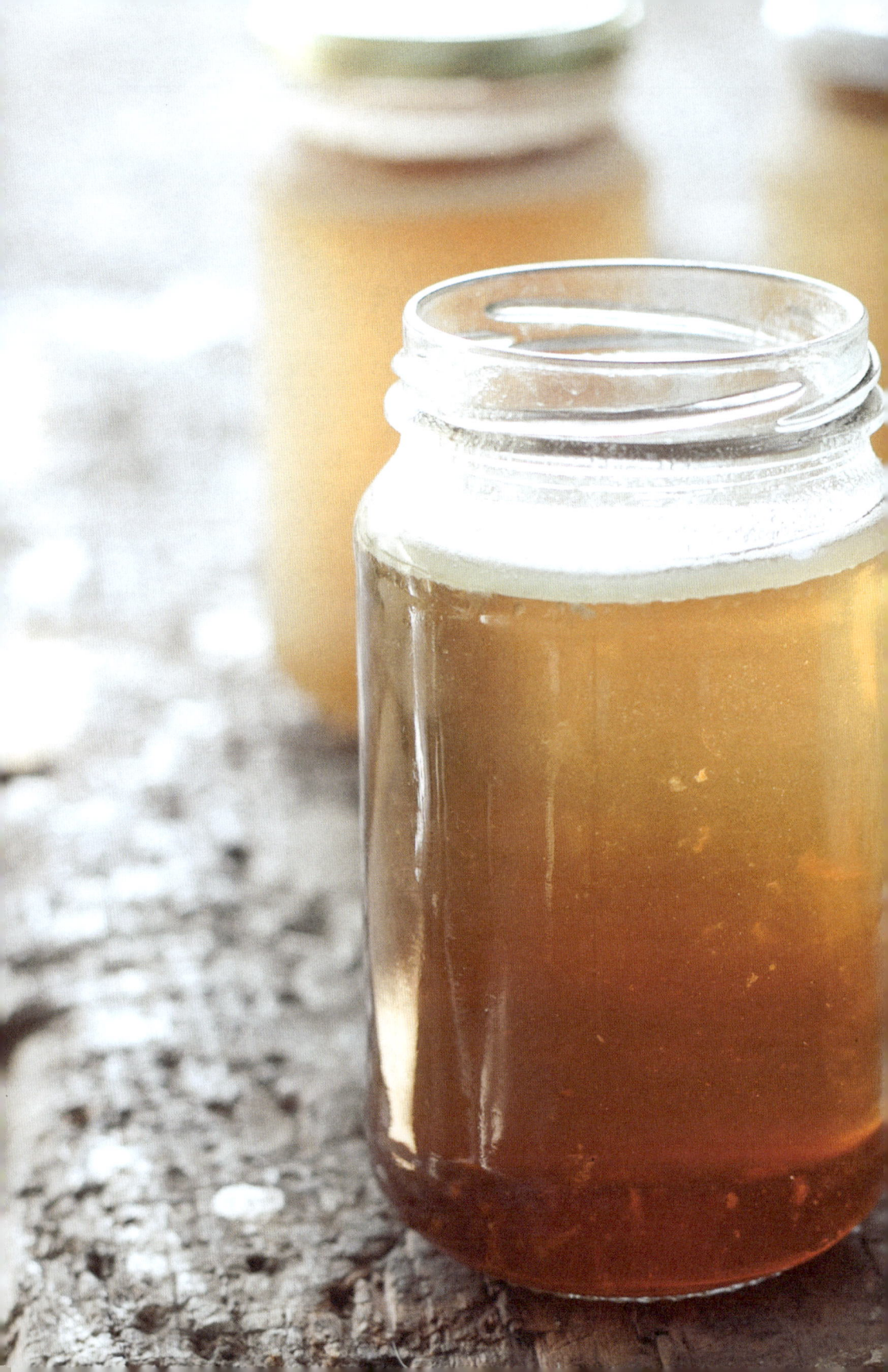

PART 1
THE TECHNICAL STUFF

The "foods" you need to quit

As the saying goes, you are what you eat. Literally, the food you consume provides the building blocks for DNA replication, new cell growth and either the maintenance of health or development of disease. The following are hardly "foods" but for the point of this discussion, the following are the key "foods" you need to quit to optimise your nutrition, and therefore health, vitality, metabolism, recovery, performance and longevity.

- Gluten
- Refined sugar
- Poor quality fats
- Poor quality dairy

Before we dive into why, consider what food was available before supermarkets or refrigerators were abundant, and before big businesses with multibillion dollar marketing budgets influenced our food choices. Food does not come in a packet or box, nor should it have a mascot. Real food comes out of the ground, off a tree or from an animal.

The point of the Real Food Athlete is to teach you what you don't need and why, and then show you how easy it is to build your plate with real food. If you are new to real food, take a deep breath and remember that Rome wasn't built in a day. Let the Real Food Athlete guide you towards making small daily changes, which will evolve into a new lifestyle in no time.

Gluten

Gluten is a protein found in wheat and its related species - rye, barley, triticale and often oats. It is responsible for the elastic texture of dough and is often used to give the final product its chewy texture and rise. Due to its complex structure, it is often used to preserve food and therefore extend its shelf life.

The problem with gluten is as a result of its particularly complex structure. Our digestive enzymes are actually unable to break the protein portion into individual (and much smaller) amino acids and it is therefore resistant to digestion. The undigested proteins then interact with our intestinal barrier and increase its permeability (intestinal permeability), to allow for the bigger molecules to pass through. While this may initially sound like a positive thing, as you may think nutrient absorption or digestion may be enhanced, the small intestine acts as our physical barrier to the outside world. When its integrity is compromised, it can no longer maintain control over what enters our bodies, and chaos occurs.

Significantly, gluten is highly inflammatory. Constant inflammation in the gut leads to intestinal permeability and potential inflammation elsewhere (or everywhere) in the body. The inflammatory effects can then appear as anything from an autoimmune disease, to chronic fatigue, allergies, arthritis, psoriasis, eczema and even brain related conditions such as depression, anxiety, bipolar disorder and schizophrenia. Inflammatory consequences are virtually unlimited and may be silent. Just because you are not experiencing specific gastrointestinal problems, does not mean you are tolerant to gluten. Even if you don't currently have an autoimmune disease, consistent exposure to gluten means you are always susceptible. Celiac disease and gluten intolerance can occur at any time. It is your environment that pulls the trigger on any genetic susceptibility.

Refined sugar

Refined sugar is the leading cause of inflammation, which can be directly linked to the longer term development of chronic disease, including diabetes, heart disease, and even cancer.

Just some of the havoc refined sugar consumption (and excess carbohydrates*) can cause in the body (and mind!):

- Insulin spikes and crashes - the blood sugar roller coaster
- Energy swings
- Cravings
- 3.30-itis
- Hanger (hunger + anger)
- A metabolism geared to sugar burning
- The requirement for 90 grams of carbohydrate/hour
- A nutritional bonk (also referred to as "hitting the wall" and nothing to do with the bedroom).

Sound familiar? Sugar will completely disrupt your fat adaptation and your ability to become a 'bonk proof' athlete. The inflammation will interfere with your recovery and subsequent performance and set you up for injuries, weight gain and the metabolic pathway to diabetes.

Gatorade, commercial sports gels and the pasta party - it's time to quit.

Carbohydrates convert to sugars and will spike your insulin and create the same negative cycle.

Poor quality fats

Seed and vegetable oils

Oils such as canola, cottonseed and grapeseed oil are high in omega-6 polyunsaturated fats (PUFAs) and therefore contain multiple double bonds in their molecular structure. Their structure can be referred to as highly 'unsaturated', which makes them incredibly unstable in the presence of heat, light or oxygen. PUFAs therefore, turn rancid and toxic at high temperatures. The longer term consequences of this include inflammation, atherogenic changes in the body and premature ageing. Please avoid margarine; keep olive oil for low temperatures and cold use only; and cook with stable saturated fats like butter, coconut oil and animal fat.

Trans fats

Here, we are referring to the artificial, synthetic, industrial or manufactured trans fats that are found in foods that use hydrogenated or partially hydrogenated vegetable fats, such as deep fried and baked foods. These foods are especially harmful as they are highly inflammatory and like refined sugar and poor quality oils, can contribute to mutagenic changes in the body and an increased chronic disease risk.

So what can I use? **Keep reading for the importance of quality fats and what you are going to use to build your plate.**

Poor quality dairy

The reality is that the majority of dairy products are highly processed via a process referred to as pasteurisation. Pasteurised dairy is subject to high temperatures to destroy impurities, which at the same time, destroys the nutritious constitutes. The truth is that the calcium actually becomes insoluble, the vitamin C is damaged, and 20% of the iodine is destroyed, just to start.

Significantly, pasteurised dairy is potentially inflammatory. Inflammation makes the body acidic, which the body then attempts to neutralize. In order to do this, calcium is leeched from the bones, causing decreased calcium levels and potentially, osteoporosis in the longer term. You have been told for decades to drink milk for strong bones, but for natural and nutrient dense options, please prioritise dark leafy greens, sardines, sesame seeds, almonds, celery, rhubarb and oranges.

In the case of skim milk, it is often fortified with powdered skim, which is liquid sprayed under heat and high pressure, a process that oxidises the cholesterol. In animal studies, oxidised cholesterol triggers a host of biological changes, leading to plaque formation in the arteries and heart disease. Low fat yoghurt is mostly high in sugar and again, devoid in nutrients due to the pastuerisation process. Throw your low fat products in the bin please.

Great alternatives to cow's milk include coconut milk and unsweetened nut milk. For more information please see your *Kitchen Makeover* (page 47).

Do I need to go Paleo?

To put it simply, dietary labels are unnecessary. When the "Paleo" diet first became popular it was quite restrictive, dogmatic and almost militant. It's great to see that this has now changed, with many influential Paleo experts now teaching moderation and non-judgement, and denouncing perfectionism. So the decision is entirely yours, just please be mindful of your approach. No one wants to be roused at the breakfast table for their avocado and feta mash.

Here are some foods you might like to include within your JERF template, that wouldn't fit a strict Paleo approach:

- **Rice malt syrup.** As it is made from rice, a grain, it is not an approved Paleo sweetener.

- **Goat's feta.** As a dairy product, it's not strictly Paleo. Goat's milk is a more tolerable form of caesin (A2). If you have a lactose intolerance, you may also find you can tolerate goat's feta, but this will come down to individual tolerance.

- **Chickpeas.** Legumes (and yes, peanuts are legumes) are not consumed on a Paleo diet, due to the supposed high phytic acid content. Paleo supporters believe this interferes with nutrient absorption, but new research now shows this may only be an issue in situations of poor gut health. Check out *The importance of gut health* (page 13) for more on this.

In summary, there are many benefits of incorporating more Paleo foods into your diet. Use the guidelines within this book to find a template that works for you and ensure it is one that is nutrient dense, sustainable and enjoyable. Food is to nourish, share and enjoy, and certainly not a quest for perfectionism.

The importance of gut health

"All disease starts in the gut." ~ Hippocrates

Gut health is the cornerstone of your health and immunity. Here is some food for thought, pun intended:

- Your gut really is your second brain, with over 95% of serotonin receptors located here.
- There is approximately 3kg of bacteria in the gut – that's more bacterial cells than human cells. Did you know that we are actually 90% bacteria? Kind of gross, but mind blowing nonetheless!

Why is gut health so important?

Gut bacteria assist in food breakdown, help produce essential nutrients and allow for greater nutrient bioavailability (via pre-digestion). Without the right balance, nutrient production, absorption, digestion and assimilation is sub-optimal. This has powerful implications for health and vitality; immunity and protection from food allergies and intolerances; cognition, memory and overall brain health; natural detoxification pathways; growth in children and adolescents; exercise performance and recovery; weight loss ability; and the list goes on…

Why is my gut health not self-regulated?

There are many reasons why we now realise that the world we live in, our choices and our behaviours are no longer supporting our gut health. Here's just a few:

- **Poor nutrition**

Prior to the recent revolution, gluten, refined sugars, refined seed oils and trans fats were everywhere. These inflammatory foods kill good gut bacteria and allow bad bacteria to thrive. Our ancestors didn't eat anything in a box, so why should we? Not to mention that our ancestors also had to ferment (i.e. preserve) their foods as they had little other choice. With the introduction of modern practices like refrigerators, canning and preservatives, the probiotic nature of traditional foods has been destroyed.

- **Stress**

We live in a modern world. We are stressed, busy and chronically tired. We are constantly exposed to heavy metals and environmental toxins and our gut health just sometimes can't compete.

- **Modern medicine**

Antibiotics, synthetic prescriptive drugs, the oral contraceptive pill (OCP)...Did you know that your gut health is passed down from your mother at conception? If your mother was ever on the OCP, it is highly likely that your gut health has been disrupted. The OCP acts like antibiotics and kills off the beneficial bacteria in the gut. If you are still taking the OCP yourself, it is time to learn another way of contraception. If you are taking the OCP to address an underlying issue, such as acne or painful periods, it is time to get to the root cause of the problem, rather than putting a bandaid over the top, and suppressing the initial problem further.

How do I know if my gut health is sub-optimal?

Honestly, you'll know. As Hippocrates said "all disease starts in the gut", so too does all health. If you are experiencing any of the following symptoms, or unusual cravings, poor bowel movements, or unexplained headaches, start healing your gut today. Burping, flatulence, bloating and excessive noises coming from your stomach are not normal. Head to *Gut Health 101* (page 68), to find out more.

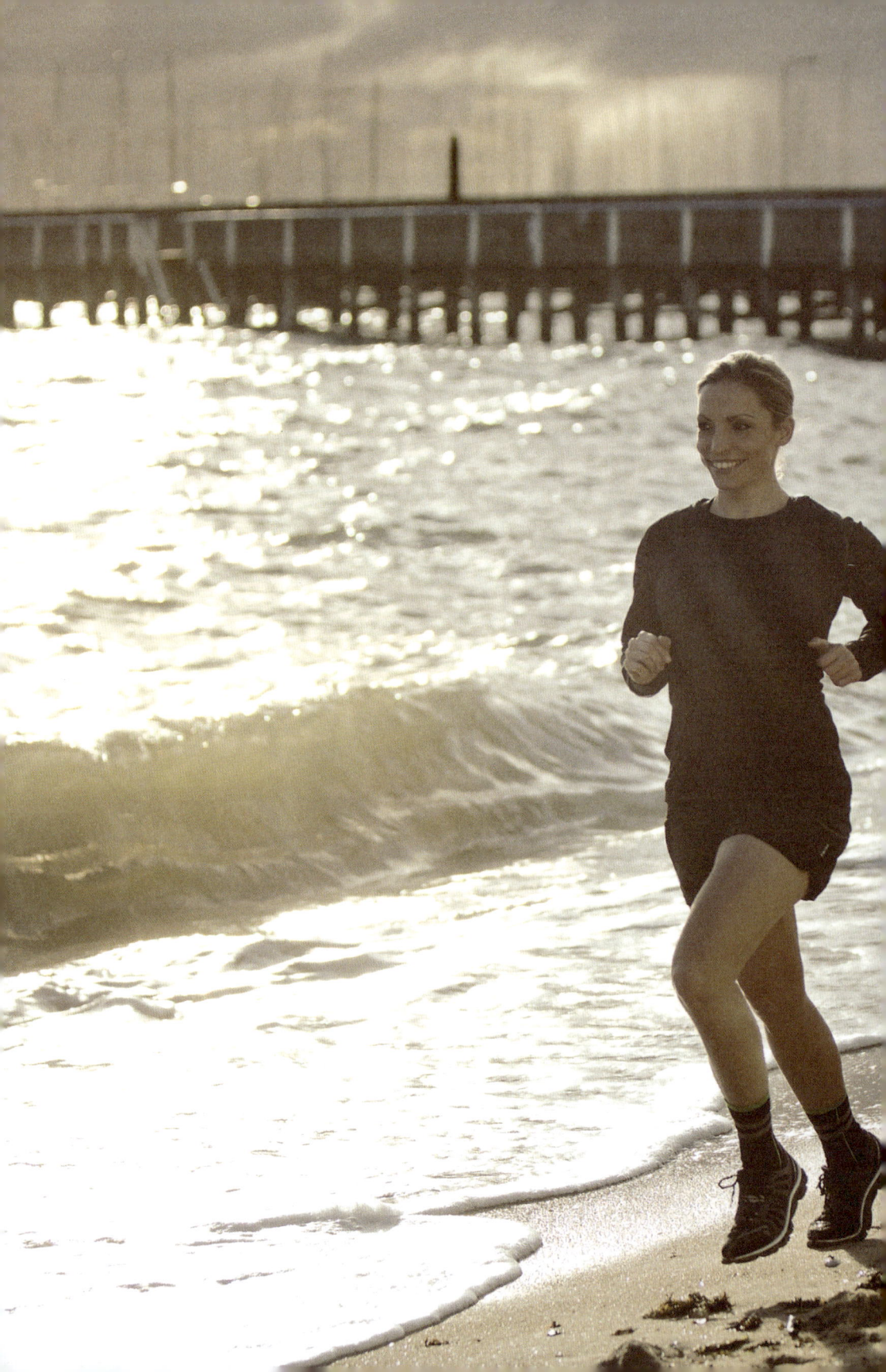

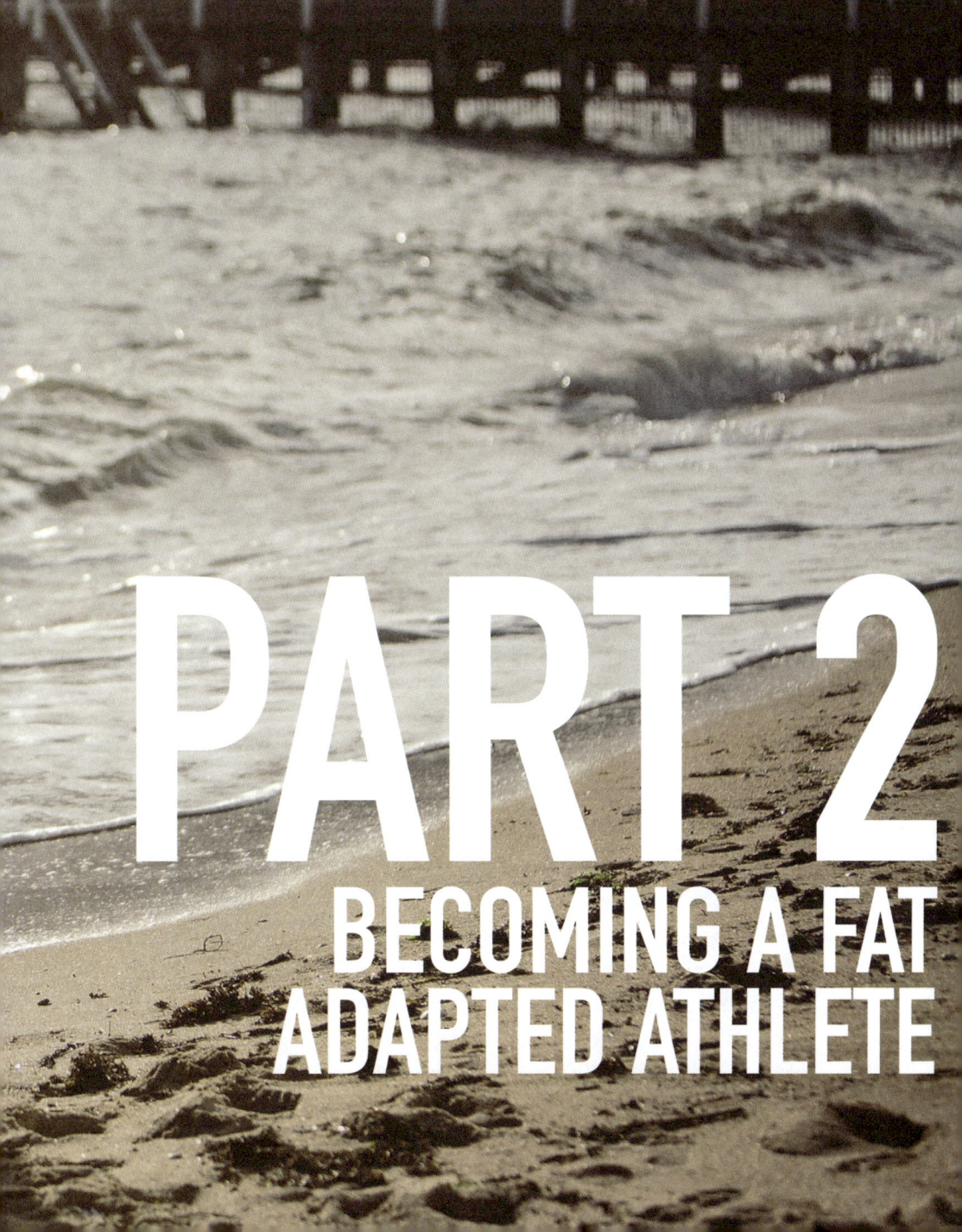

Fat Adaptation 101

Fat adaptation is the metabolic reorchestration from a predominant fuel source of glucose to a predominant fuel source of fat.

This is the normal, preferred metabolic state of the human. Before the food pyramid created the obesity epidemic, humans were in a constant yearly cycle of fat adaptation, based on factors such location, climate, season and food supply.

Consider the following:

- Fat adaptation means you can effectively burn stored fat for energy throughout the day. Even the leanest person who weighs 60kg with 10% body fat, has 6kg of fat or 6000g, which at 9 calories/gram is 54,000 calories to potentially access.
- Fat adaptation also means you can rely more on fat for energy during exercise. This offers a glycogen sparing effect, so this fuel (carbohydrate stored in the muscle) is available to support high intensity exercise, where it is most required.
- For endurance athletes, this is most significant. A simple equation to consider (using round numbers): even a well trained 'sugar burning' athlete with 2000 calories of muscle glycogen stored, who burns 1000 calories/hour, will obviously run out of fuel at beyond two hours. Even if the athlete was able to consume 300 calories/hour, there's still a 700-calorie

deficit. The inability to tap into fat reserves is what causes a 'nutritional bonk' or 'hitting the wall'. If you're an endurance athlete whose splits just get slower and slower during a marathon off the bike or ultra marathon, you need to work on your fat adaptation so you essentially never run out of fuel.

The benefits of fat adaptation

1. **Metabolic flexibility.** Metabolic flexibility is the capacity to adapt fuel oxidation to fuel availability. The advantage of being a fat burner is that you can still burn glucose when necessary and/or available, but you have an almost unlimited reserve of fuel available from fat. Sugar burners only have one fuel option - they can't effectively access dietary fat for energy, and as a result, more fat is stored than burned.

2. **Glycogen sparing.** Carbohydrates are stored in the muscle as glycogen but even a well-trained athlete is capped at 2000 calories. Sugar burners rely significantly on this energy source and essentially waste their glycogen on efforts that fat should be able to power. Fat burners can preserve muscle glycogen for when it is most required, such as the back end of a training session or competition, and outperform their sugar-burning counterparts any day of the week.

3. **Improved performance.** The burning of carbohydrates results in the production of lactic acid and reactive oxygen species, which create oxidative damage that your body must mop up using antioxidants. Fats burn "clean" however, producing only carbon dioxide and water, allowing oxidative damage to be avoided, and energy and resources to be prioritised to the recovery process. Faster recovery means you can get back

out there and train better the next day, and for the entire season.

4. **Improved recovery.** In addition to removing the constant oxidative damage from relying on carbohydrates as a predominant fuel, processed food and refined sugars are highly inflammatory. Inflammation is extremely detrimental to your recovery and subsequent performance, so removing these foods is key.

5. **Injury prevention.** Promoting an anti-inflammatory environment prevents inflammation associated injuries. If you want to avoid falling down this hole, focus on burning a clean fuel during training or racing, and therefore, your nutrition choices meal-to-meal.

6. **Enhanced immunity.** Your gut contains 80% of your immune system, so it's clear that what you put in your mouth has a direct influence on your immunity. By removing refined sugar, gluten, poor quality fats and poor quality dairy, you are providing the essential building blocks of a healthy immune system. To this we add a gut health practice, which you can read about on page 68.

7. **Goal weight becomes easy to maintain.** As a fat burner you can effectively access dietary fat for energy and as a result, less fat is stored. Furthermore, postprandial fat oxidation is increased, and again, less dietary fat is stored in adipose tissue. By burning fat efficiently, you can achieve your goal weight without starvation, hunger, counting calories or the metabolic disruption that comes with a calorie-restricted approach.

8. **A more efficient metabolism day-to-day.** With the increased ability to oxidise dietary fat for energy, you no longer need

to snack every two hours. This creates a freedom from food and your appetite, controls your energy and moods, and allows for digestive ease. Conversely, sugar burners are "hangry" (hunger + angry), and with the age-related decrease in glucose tolerance, often on the pathway to pre-diabetes.

9. **A more efficient metabolism in training and racing.** When you can use fat as a predominant fuel, you direct energy outwards to working heart, muscle and lungs, rather than inwards to digestion. Metabolic flexibility will completely change your fuelling requirements and you will no longer need 60-90 grams of carbohydrates per hour in training. You should perform consistently and finish stronger, provided your training has been optimal. You essentially become "bonk proof".

10. **Avoidance of gastro-intestinal (GI) distress.** Being fat adapted and no longer consuming mass amounts of carbohydrates (particularly fructose) during training and racing significantly decreases the likelihood of GI distress. Unlike glucose, fructose is not absorbed from the intestine but must be transported by the blood to the liver where it is converted to glucose. It is absorbed by the intestines more slowly, which in many athletes can cause cramping and diarrhoea, especially with the high doses that are required by sugar-burning athletes.

11. **Logistical ease on race day.** With decreased fuelling requirements, your bike does not look like a buffet and you don't need to rely on special needs. Racing becomes stress-free, as you now only need a small amount of exogenous fuel to stoke the fire that is your fat oxidation. More on this to come.

12. **Increased athletic longevity.** As sugar is highly inflammatory, a real food approach is vital if you want to prevent injuries, improve your health markers and lower your risk of chronic disease. Eating well and optimising your metabolism means you perform better, remain lean, and stay metabolically healthy, as you go up in age group.

How to get there

The two basic strategies are as follows:

- A low carbohydrate high fat (LCHF) approach is particularly useful in the 'off-season' to enhance fat adaptation, as it decreases your physiology of being a sugar burner (because of a high carbohydrate intake) and allows for five or more hours between meals based on the satiety and blood sugar response it creates. This allows for metabolic efficiency on a day-to-day basis. A very general guide is a total intake of 15% carbohydrates, 20% protein, and 65% good fats per day.

- The second is fasted training, or training empty. When practised in training (ideally in the off-season) for 8-12 weeks, this enhances fat utilisation and decreases reliance on exogenous fuel sources (e.g. gels). Start with lower intensity sessions of 60-90 minutes in duration. As your fat adaptation progresses, gradually extend this to two or two-and-a-half hours. Beyond this is often unnecessary in order to avoid catabolism (muscle breakdown) that can occur over extended durations.

The metabolic grey zone

Athletes who are complete sugar burners transitioning to LCHF may experience the 'metabolic grey zone'. No carbohydrates coming in and an inability to burn fat, means the overall energy provision feels low, even in the case of higher than normal calories. Initially this can contribute to fatigue, hunger, and poor performance. The good news is that most athletes only experience this for 3-4 days. It can however last for a couple of weeks and why the best time to start is in the off season or when training can be adapted accordingly.

After this initial phase there are so many benefits. The biggest difference experienced day-to-day is satiety, shifting from insatiable hunger, snacking every two hours to being well fuelled with four, five or more hours in between meals. The case of hangry (hunger + angry) is a thing of the past and it's quite life changing for most. And it's this satiety that keeps the fat adaptation continuing - when you don't need to eat for five hours you open up a huge fat burning opportunity between meals.

Fuelling for training and racing

Firstly, prioritise what is known as 'train low'. This means starting your sessions fasted, and experimenting with how much, or how little fuel you need per hour. If you're just commencing fat adaptation, start with 30-45 grams/hour. If you've been following a traditional sports nutrition model and working off 90 grams/hour then you will need to scale back slowly. The key indicators to track are energy, digestion, performance and recovery. It is important to remember that nutrition is extremely relative and it is your responsibility to get out in the field and test a number of potential strategies that can then be looked at for race day.

Many athletes are surprised to hear this, but you can apply fasted principles on race morning, as although an Ironman is a nine or even 17-hour day, fuelling can begin as early as heart rate stabilisation on the bike. It's therefore, on average, a 60-90 minute fasted session, depending on how fast you swim. Your muscle glycogen levels should be full (provided you've refuelled and tapered well) and only your liver glycogen would have depleted slightly over night, making it unnecessary for more carbohydrates at this time. It may sound unconventional that you don't need breakfast or a gel pre-Ironman, but with optimum fat adaptation it is more than possible.

A caveat to this is if you are hungry and/or prefer to eat on race day (and have practiced this in training) then by all means eat, but keep it to low carb, good fats and moderate protein, such as bacon and eggs or a smoothie you could even prepare the night before. Waking up three hours earlier than you need to, in order to eat your carbohydrate-rich meal, creates not only a logistical nightmare, but sets up the cycle for increased carbohydrate requirements, most likely and inconveniently when you're face down in a body of water.

Race day fuelling

On race day, you essentially have two choices:

1. Use your 'train low' fuelling strategy that you refined during training. The strategic use of carbohydrates on race day is essential for high intensity and for the ability to access your fat reserves; or

2. What is referred to as 'race high', or a higher carbohydrate gram/hour intake. When you're fat adapted, you utilise the carbohydrates far more efficiently, and in general, will still be using less than a traditional sports nutrition model. On race day this is beneficial from both a digestive and logistical sense. The amount you need is of course extremely relative, and you would have determined this during training. You should only need a handful of trial runs to not detract from your fat adaptation.

Post-training/Refuelling

This is where nutrient timing is important. You need smaller amounts (30-45 grams) of carbohydrates post-training for muscle glycogen replenishment (nutrient timing). Scale this based on session intensity and subsequent recovery and performance. For example, if you start with 30 grams post training and your recovery is not optimal in the days following, increase to 45 grams after a similar session and compare. Being an intuitive athlete is important here.

A caveat here is a very well fat adapted athlete who can intuitively decide that carbohydrates are not required after a particular low intensity session. Please be mindful not to dig yourself into thyroid dysfunction with an excessively low carbohydrate approach, and always exercise caution if you take this approach. It's not about eliminating or demonising carbohydrates, it's about the strategic use. Read that again.

Common mistakes to avoid

- The number one barrier to fat adaptation is stress. A very short physiology lesson: in situations of stress our adrenal glands produce the hormone cortisol (and adrenaline). This is part of our 'flight or fight' response and is necessary to human optimal function and survival. The role of cortisol is to stimulate the liver to release glucose into the blood, so that in the caveman days, we were supplied with an immediate source of fuel to help us run away from or defend ourselves against predators. In modern days, where stress is chronic and cortisol levels are therefore consistently elevated, this excess glucose inhibits fat utilisation. Longer term, chronic cortisol production overworks the adrenal glands and can end up as adrenal fatigue. This is not to be taken lightly.

- Secondly, a common mistake is inefficient nutrient timing. Remember, nutrient timing is the consumption of real food-based carbohydrates in the post-training window. This is particularly important after high intensity exercise, as muscle glycogen has been depleted. But as a society we are used to consuming carbohydrates with every meal and the adjustment away from this can be challenging for some (see *The metabolic grey zone* on page 24). It's important to remember that carbohydrates in excess will spike the hormone insulin, which immediately shuts off fat burning. Carbohydrate intake needs to be managed relatively closely in the initial phases but the good news is that once the metabolic reorchestration takes place, most athletes can stay fat adapted on far more than 15% carbohydrate.

- Thirdly, fat phobia. Our calorie counting and low-fat ways of the past can trip a lot of athletes up. You are now free to eat butter, avocado and full fat foods, but you may be still afraid of these foods. It is extremely important to note that you cannot cut carbs and fat at the same time and remember on LCHF, our fat intake is over 60% of our daily intake. If you're hungry within 4 hours of eating, add more fat and watch your satiety extend.

- Another common mistake is excess protein. Excess protein is converted to glucose via gluconeogenesis, which interferes with blood sugar control and can promote high insulin. As we discussed, this shuts off fat burning. For most, an intake of 20% protein is more that enough. So on a 1700-calorie day, this is only 85 grams. Even a male eating 3000 calories, needs less than 150 grams of protein per day.

- And lastly, low salt intake. The fear that salt with give you high blood pressure and kill you is another dogma-based myth of the last five decades. As you become fat adapted your salt requirements increase dramatically, so please add good quality salt (e.g. Himalayan) liberally to your meals to maintain an optimum blood volume. Athletes who experience poor performance or fatigue beyond their initial adaptation phase, must test a higher salt intake and their physiological response to this.

Am I a fat burner?

Metabolic Efficiency Testing (MET)

A Metabolic Efficiency Test (MET) is a great way to test your current fat burning ability, as it measures both your aerobic fitness and your fuel utilisation at varying exercise intensities. It will provide tangible evidence of where you are starting from, and a good indication of your metabolic reorchestration (from a preferential fuel of sugar to fat) after 8-12 weeks of fat adaptation.

The key data you will obtain is:
- VO_{2max} ml/kg/min - a measure of the maximum volume of oxygen that an athlete can use; indicative of aerobic fitness. It is measured in millilitres per kilogram of body weight per minute (ml/kg/min).
- Respiratory quotient (RQ) - the ratio of carbon dioxide you produce to oxygen you consume. An RQ of 1.0+ indicates you are a full sugar burner and an RQ of 0.7 indicates full fat burning. Somewhere around 0.8 means you're fairly well fat adapted, where the closer to 1 you get, the more of a sugar burner you are.
- Crossover point (COP): this is the heart rate at which a higher carbohydrate contribution occurs, at an RQ of approximately 0.85. The higher your heart rate at the COP and the further the COP moves to the right, the more advantageous this is. Athletes should train under their COP to promote fat oxidation and expect to see substantial shifts with fat adaptation.
- Metabolic data - carbohydrate grams per hour and fat grams

per hour burnt at varying intensities, power and/or %VO_2*. This data is most beneficial for developing or confirming your fuelling plan.

A MET can be obtained via your local Exercise Physiologist and costs $200-300.

For a more affordable approach, contact the Human Movement/ Sports Science Department of your local university and sign yourself up as a research subject.

*Please check that this particular data is obtained prior to commencing your test as not all laboratories provide the same information.

Your 12-week timeline

MET > 8-12 weeks > MET > adjustment, if required

Key points during the 8-12 weeks:

- 2/1/2 with nutrient timing (page 41-43)

- 15/20/65 (page 24)

- 3 meals/day

- Fasted training

- Natural fuelling (page 191-212)

When is the ideal time to start?

It depends. If you're looking to dial in your nutrition for fat adaptation, a minimum of 8 weeks will yield the best results. If you're coming from a traditional sports nutrition model (i.e. high carbohydrate), your key sessions may be comprised if major changes are made too close to race day.

The ideal time to start working on your metabolic efficiency is post-race, when training volume is low, stress management can be prioritised, and time can be allocated to food preparation and the development of your new routine.

If you are well on your way and just need to fine tune things, then 4-6 weeks will work. The main thing to consider from a fuelling perspective is key sessions to trial strategies in, in order to replicate race day as closely as possible. The number one rule in racing is nothing new happens on race day.

What about strength athletes?

Something to consider is that for most of human existence, humans ate concentrated sources of carbohydrates three to five times a year. When fruit was ripe or honey was available our ancestors perhaps over-consumed short term, but importantly, carbohydrates were not consumed three to five times per day, week after week or decade after decade. For the majority of the year our ancestors consumed a diet rich in animal fats, and thrived.

Even if you are lifting PBs all week, your carbohydrate storage is capped. You cannot keep consuming carbohydrates and expect your body to adapt to storing more. Once a sink is full, it's full. If you can tap into fat for energy however, the preservation of muscle glycogen is the key to your performance. The longer you can power your efforts on fat, the more you can save glycogen for the later, more intense efforts, like the back end of a competition or training session.

One caveat to our nutritional recommendations is that you may benefit from a small portion of carbohydrate pre-training, taking you up to three meals and one snack per day. This applies predominately to high-intensity sessions or competition. Once you are metabolically flexible this won't be detrimental to your fat oxidation, but it will allow your body to continue to access fat and provide glucose for where it is most required.

Remember that "training low" will continue to enhance your fat oxidation and provide the significant short and long-term benefits associated with this. Go back to page 26 for a quick recap.

How much?

The more fat adapted you are, the less you will need. As always, start with one portion or 30 grams of carbohydrates and scale upwards only if required. You will need to individually test your timing pre-training, based on digestive ease and performance and recovery outcomes.

Please see page 26 for carbohydrate portion recommendations.

What about yoga?

Being a fat adapted yogi will allow you to finish a class strong and optimise your performance and recovery day-to-day and week-to-week. Controlling your metabolism is essential to get or stay lean, prevent injuries and be in charge of your long-term health.

Nutrient timing is a fantastic way to enjoy good quality carbohydrates, with the rest of your day based on our principles of 2/1/2. Pre-training recommendations do not apply, as it is always best to practice yoga on an empty stomach. Many yogis are already well on their way to fat adaptation as they have not been subject to the carbohydrate-driven and dogmatic nutritional recommendations of the endurance world.

If you enjoy hot yoga, please be mindful that your hydration requirements increase relative to your output. This can easily be managed with filtered water and electrolytes from fresh lemon (our highest electrolyte containing fruit) and a pinch of Himalayan salt. Please be mindful that each 200ml bottle of coconut water contains 15 grams of sugar, so this should be allocated to intense and hot sessions only. If you do select coconut water post-yoga, please factor this in to the total volume of carbohydrates consumed in this window.

It is important to note that if you consume excess carbohydrate post-training you will not obtain the satiety benefits of our real food approach. When your meal provides five or more hours of satiety, you know you have your personalised balance of macronutrients right.

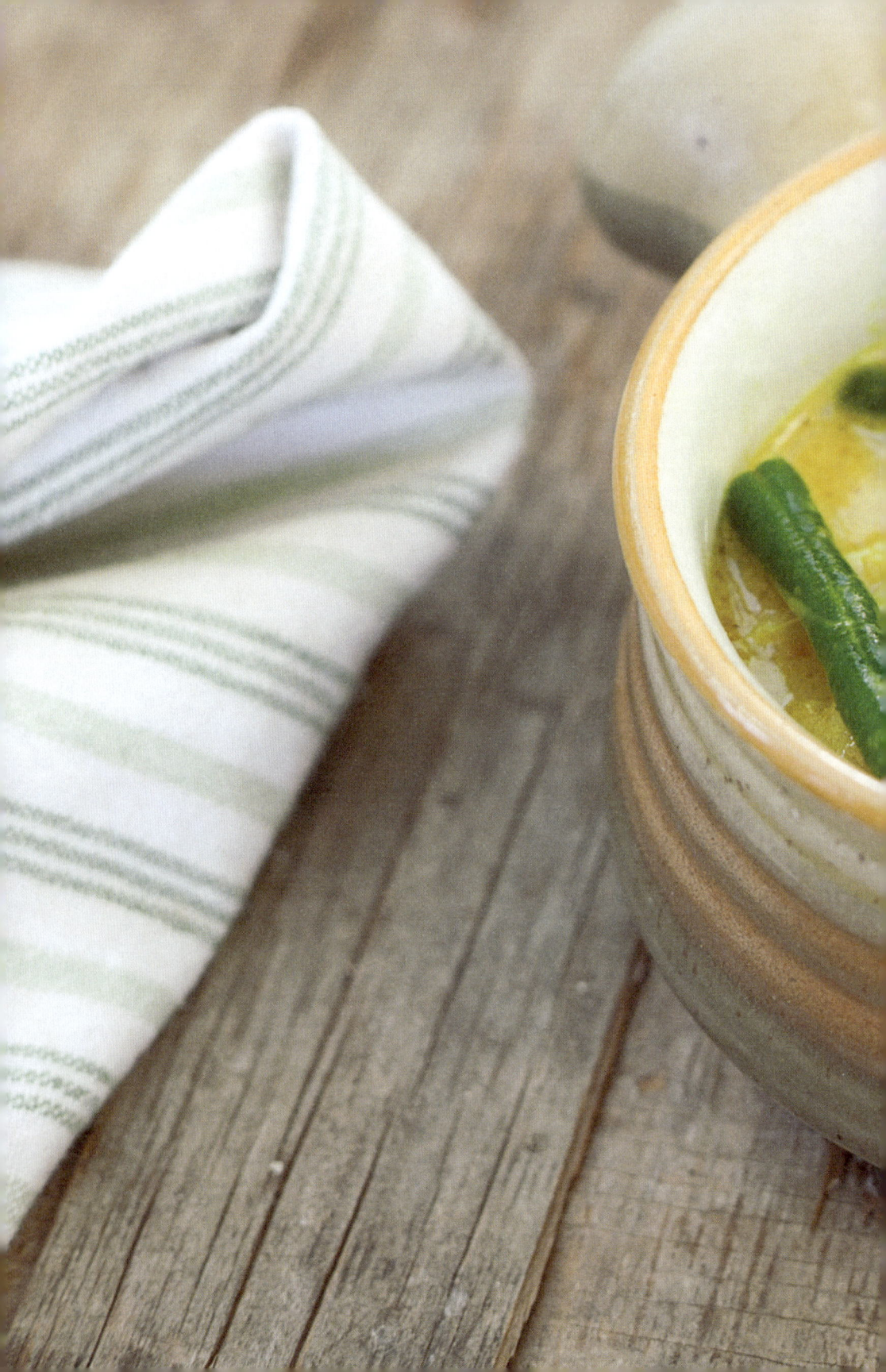

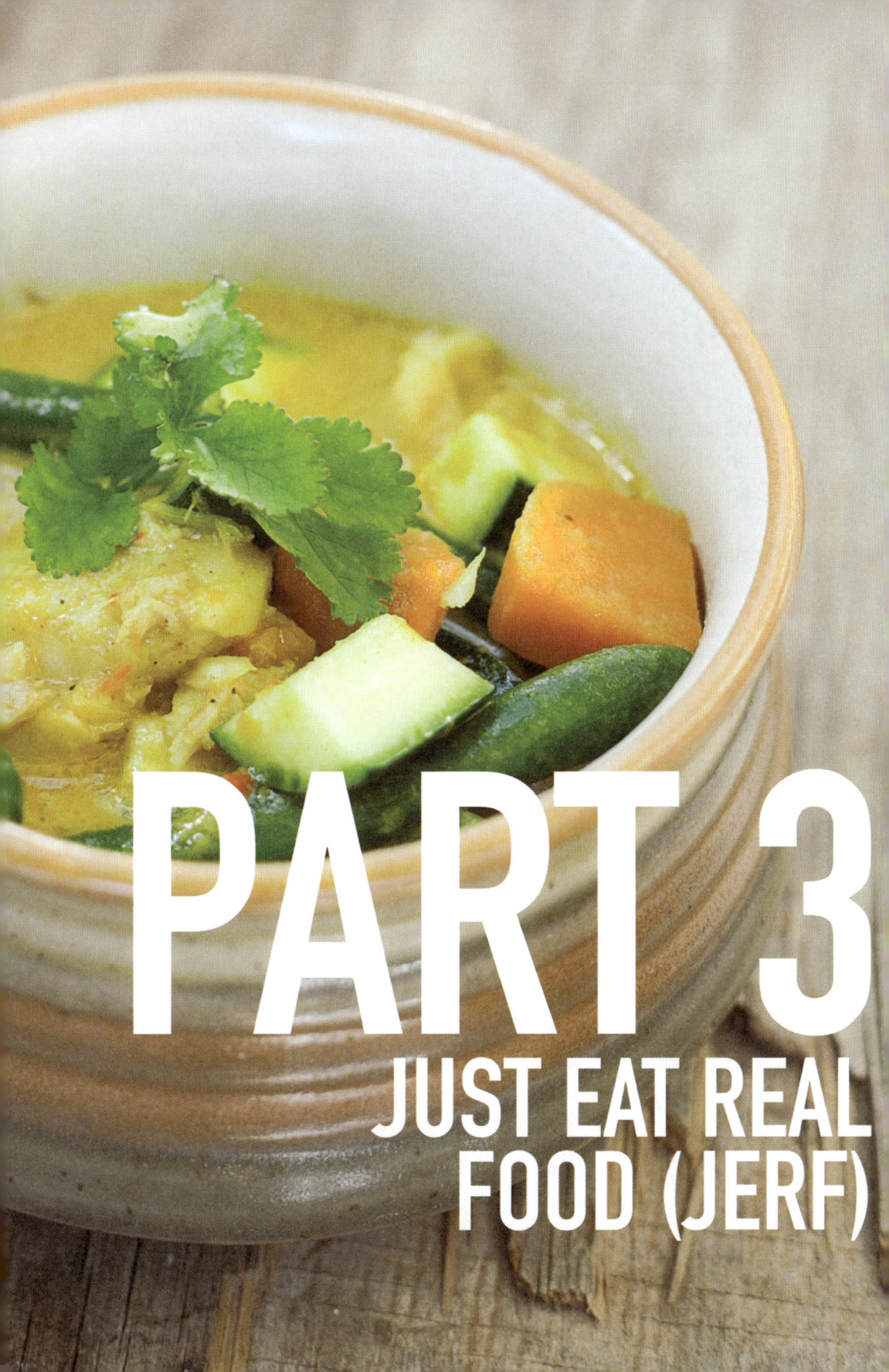

PART 3

JUST EAT REAL FOOD (JERF)

JERF

- **What?** Food that comes out of the ground, off a tree or from an animal is always the most nutrient dense and whole food source of nutrition.

- **Why?** An anti-inflammatory approach free of gluten, refined sugars, poor quality fats and poor quality dairy will optimise your health, energy levels, hormones, performance, recovery and athletic longevity.

- **How?** The biggest change you can make to improve your health is to significantly reduce or eliminate your packaged food consumption.

Whether your goal is to become a fat adapted athlete, healthier, happier, or lean, JERF is for you.

How to build your plate

Real food is as simple as 2/1/2. To build your plate:

- Start with two (2) cups of predominately non-starchy vegetables with each meal.

- Combine one (1) serve of protein, such as a palm-size piece of meat or fish, or three eggs.

- Add two (2) portions of good fats, such as half an avocado and 30g of butter; or 30ml of olive oil and a handful of nuts and seeds.

- Complex/starchy carbohydrates are then added post training (nutrient timing) at one (1) portion.

2/1/2

* Non-starchy vegetables - 2 cups with every meal

- Asparagus
- Leek
- Onion
- Broccoli
- Brussels sprouts
- Pumpkin
- Alfalfa
- Zucchini
- Celery
- Cauliflower
- Bok choy
- Artichoke
- Spinach
- Lettuce
- Kale
- Capsicum
- Mushrooms
- Eggplant
- Cucumber
- Squash
- Cabbage
- Tomato
- Carrots
- Fennel

Please note: this list is not exhaustive. Beans, snow peas and peas are legumes and best on occasions only. Please avoid corn as it is a grain.

* Protein - 1 portion with every meal

1 palm-size piece of meat/fish/chicken/beef/lamb or approximately 100g

1 small can tuna, salmon or sardines

2 slices bacon

3 eggs

1 scoop (30g) quality protein powder such as Bare Blends

* Fats - 2 portions with every meal

½ avocado

30g grass-fed butter

30g nuts (limit cashews due to high carbohydrate content; peanuts are legumes)

30ml flaxseed/coconut/macadamia/extra virgin olive oil

100ml coconut cream

Please note: One (1) serve of grass fed meats and free range eggs also provide approximately half (0.5) a serve of good fats.

*Complex/starchy carbohydrates (Post-training)

1 piece of fruit (e.g. banana, apple, orange)

½ cup sweet potato, potato, beetroot

½ cup quinoa, buckwheat, basmati rice (cooked)

2 slices gluten free bread*

*Bread is obviously not 'JERF', but if you choose to eat it occasionally, then it forms a part of the balanced approach we are striving for. Where possible, ensure quality by making a selection from your local health food store.

Examples

2/1/2 is as simple as:

- A three-egg omelette with spinach, tomato and mushroom, served with half an avocado.

- A smoothie including avocado, coconut cream, protein powder and spinach.

- A salad of spinach, tomato, capsicum, walnuts, goat's feta and tuna, topped with an olive oil and apple cider vinegar dressing.

- A salmon fillet served with steamed greens topped with grass-fed butter and Himalayan salt. After an intense session add 1/2 cup sweet potato chips.

Carbs, carbs, carbs!

We have discussed the importance of controlling your carbohydrate to accelerate fat adaptation. Here's what you can eat:

- Real food carbohydrates are always preferential to packaged wholegrains and cereals.

- Prioritise starchy vegetables and fruit. Quinoa and rice are fine once or twice a week.

- Eat these predominately in your post-training meal, to top up muscle glycogen and accelerate your recovery and subsequent performance goals.

This provides the best of both worlds - a fat adapted metabolism with enhanced recovery and subsequent performance. Examples include half a banana with your breakfast or half cup of sweet potato with dinner after an evening run.

How much carbohydrate do I need?

The answer is, it depends.

- A 'metabolically healthy' endurance athlete might need 200 grams of carbohydrate per day.

- A sedentary person will most likely need <100 grams of carbohydrate per day.

- Diabetics often need <25 grams of carbohydrate per day.

Using blood tests to determine what you really need

The two most common fasting blood markers you can use to assist are:

- Glycated hemoglobin - HbA1C (%): ideal <5.3%

- Blood glucose level (BGL): ideal <5.0 mmol/L

The higher your levels, the more carbohydrate resistant you are, and the less you should consume.

For help with your macronutrient profile, please read *"Do you need personalised support with your real food journey?"* on page 225.

Kitchen makeover

Pantry basics

Stock your kitchen with these staples first, and getting started will be easy.

- Nut milk

- Almond flour

- Coconut flour

- Raw cacao

- Coconut oil

- Rice malt syrup

- Quinoa

Nut milk

Ingredients
- 1 cup nuts (e.g. almonds, walnuts, cashews, macadamia or unsweetened coconut flakes)
- 5 cups water
- 1 tablespoon Pure Harvest organic rice malt syrup
- 1 tablespoon cinnamon

Method
1. Soak your choice of nut for at least six hours in one cup of water.
2. Drain and rinse nuts and blend with four cups of water.
3. Add the rice malt syrup and cinnamon and blend again.
4. Pour through a strainer into a large bowl.
5. Pour into a tightly sealed bottle and store in the fridge for up to a week.
6. Save your pulp – simply bake in an oven on a very low heat for 3 hours, stirring regularly and voila, you have nut milk. You may need to blend it to make muffins, but for Chocolate Brownie Bites the extra crunch is just perfect.

Not ready to make your own?

Pure Harvest have a fantastic unsweetened almond milk and the divine CocoQuench. For more information and stockists, please visit www.pureharvest.com.au.

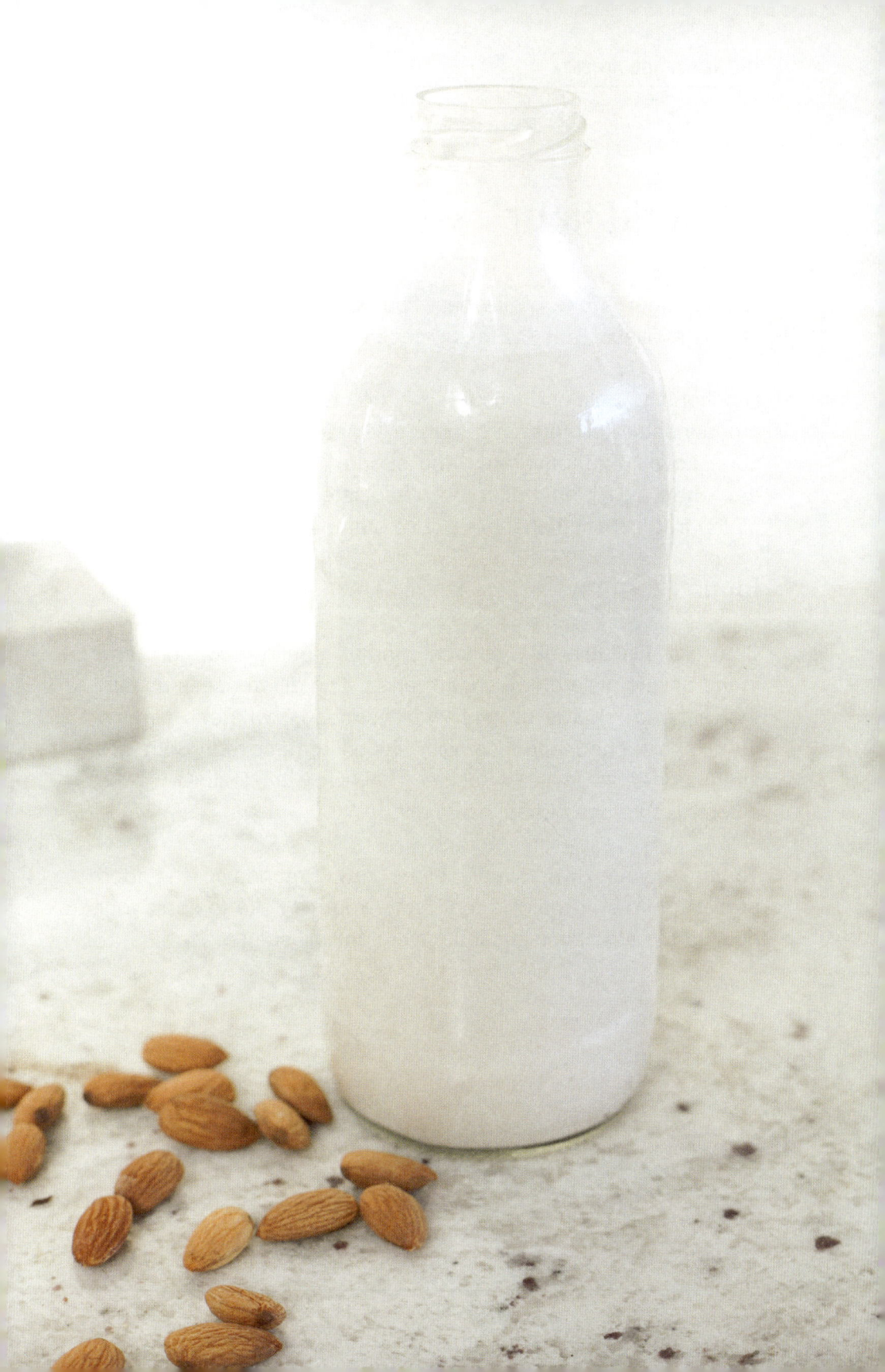

Almond flour

Almond flour is one of the best flour substitutes available. It is readily available, easy to make, cook with, and delicious.

Nutritionally, almond flour is full of our heart-healthy monounsaturated fats, and high in vitamin E, magnesium and fibre. Low in carbohydrates and sugars – it's perfect to avoid the 'wheat belly', or 'muffin top', associated with some common gluten free substitutions, like potato starch and corn starch.

Flour vs. meal

Both are available at your local market, health food store and in the baking aisle of the supermarket. The difference is usually that almond meal is ground whole almonds, whereas almond flour is blanched almonds with the skin removed. Both are interchangeable in most recipes, however the texture will be different, so please keep this in mind.

To make your own, simply blend raw almonds in the food processor. Yes, it really is that easy. You may like to soak your nuts first to assist in digestion. Overnight will suffice.

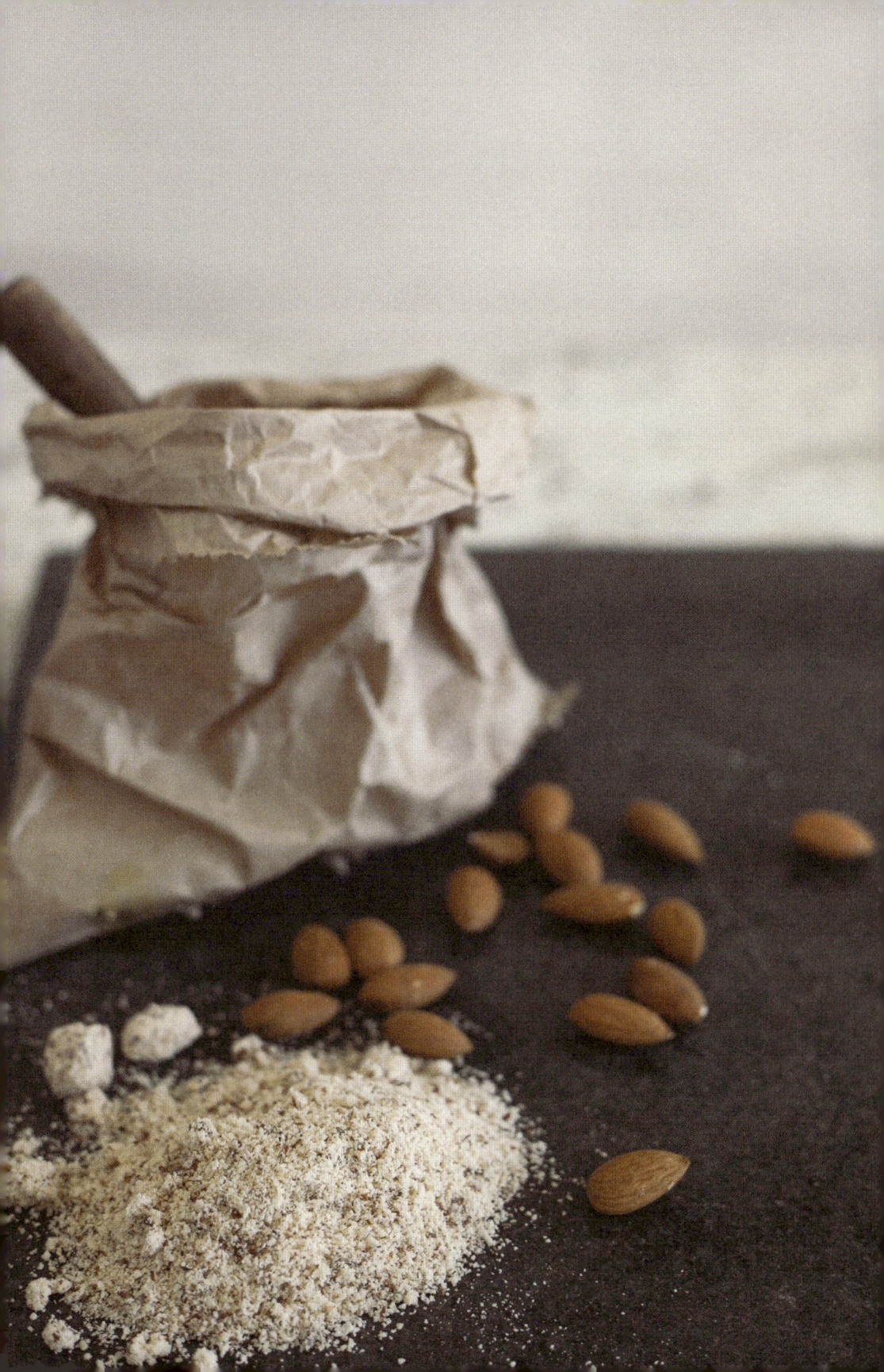

Coconut flour

Coconut flour is a must-have addition to your pantry. It is not only gluten free, grain free and low carbohydrate, but also extremely nutritious. Here's why:

- Coconut flour is 14% coconut oil, a medium chain triglyceride (MCT) that is easily digested and readily absorbed by the liver. MCTs are used as a direct source of energy by our brains and muscles rather than for fat storage (which is what happens when you consume trans fats, amongst other things). Studies show that the consumption of coconut oil can assist in calorie burning, fat oxidation and reduced food intake, and as a result, weight loss.

- Coconut flour is made up of 58% dietary fibre, and is therefore fantastic for blood sugar control, satiety and curbing cravings, all of which are essential for weight management. It is one of the biggest nutrition myths that wholegrains and cereals are required for fibre, when fruit and vegetables are the highest sources of fibre known to man.

- Coconut flour is rich in protein – great for satiety, blood sugar control, immunity and recovery from exercise, just to start.

- Coconut flour contains manganese, a vitamin that is essential for the thyroid gland, which is the regulator of our metabolism, growth and energy expenditure.

Coconut flour: tips and tricks

- Due to its density, unfortunately you cannot simply substitute coconut flour for other flours. A useful guide is to start with one third of a cup for every cup of 'normal' flour.

- Coconut flour and almond flour work really well together. If the density of coconut flour on its own is not to your liking, you may like to modify with half a cup of each. Adding a small amount to your favourite recipe is a great place to start, and should not change the liquid requirements or texture too much.

- Coconut flour is not just for sweet treats. It makes a great Gluten Free Chicken Schnitz or can be used as a breadcrumb replacement for coating meatballs. It does have a sweeter flavour than conventional flours though, so keep that in mind when cooking for others.

- Coconut flour is one of the more expensive flours, so the solution is to shop online or make your own using unsweetened coconut flakes and water. Use the nut milk recipe (page 48) as a guide.

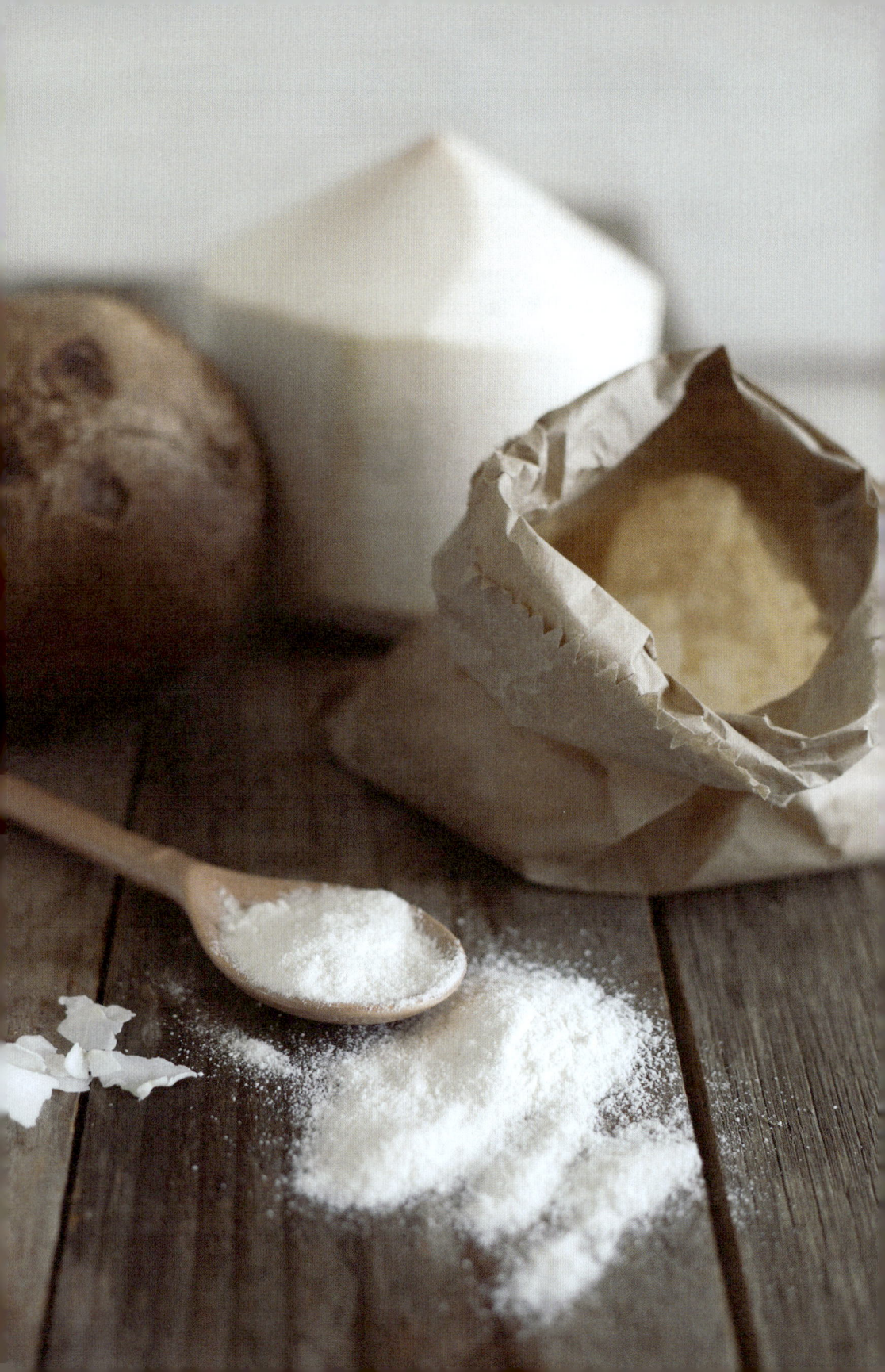

Raw cacao

Raw cacao is nature's super bean. Due to its extremely high ORAC score (a measure of antioxidant quantity), it is actually classed as a 'super-antioxidant' and therefore helps to prevent cellular damage, protect the heart, and naturally fight the ageing process.

Cacao is also a great source of flavonoids, essential fatty acids and magnesium – all of which help with metabolism, premenstrual symptoms, heart function, blood pressure and lowering chronic disease risk. Raw cacao contains naturally occurring theobromine, which acts as a mild, non-addictive stimulant that some believe can treat depression. Studies show that theobromine assists the brain to produce more anandamide, a 'feel good' neurotransmitter.

A side note: cacao is not the same as cocoa (which is highly processed and low in nutrition), and is always best in its raw form, without the added sugar that most commercial chocolates contain. Opt for 85% dark chocolate when you can, and try this Natural Hot Chocolate to assist with sugar cravings and to aid satiety after a meal.

Natural Hot Chocolate

Ingredients
- 1 teaspoon raw cacao
- 100ml unsweetened nut milk
- 1 cup boiled water
- 1 teaspoon Pure Harvest organic rice malt syrup (optional)

Method
1. Add cacao to a large mug, add boiled water and stir well.
2. Top with milk and for a little sweetness, rice malt syrup.

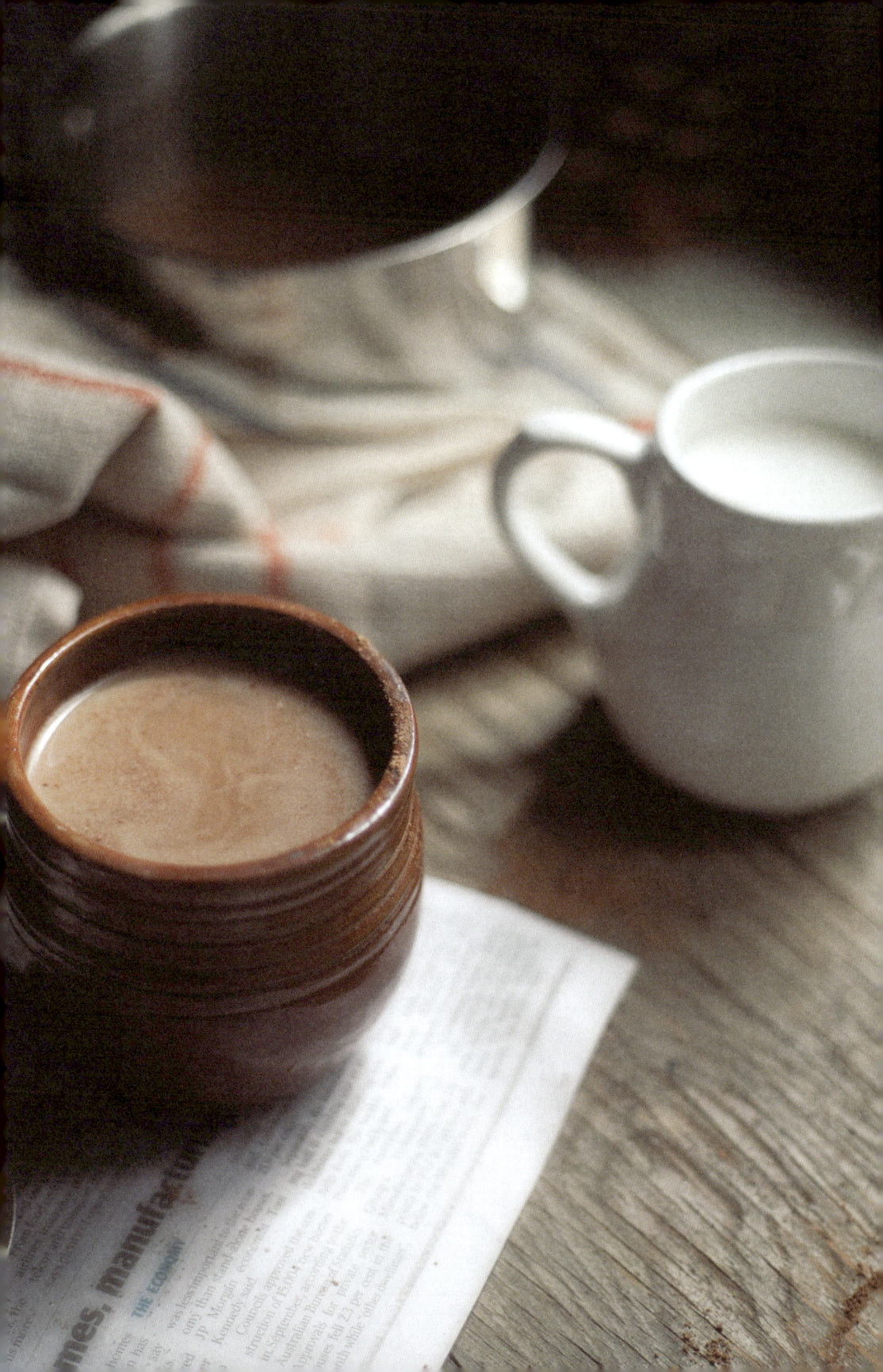

Coconut oil

Coconut oil has a high saturated fat content and more specifically, is high (66%) in MCTs. In contrast to long chain triglycerides, MCTs are easily digested and readily absorbed by the liver, and are therefore a direct source of energy. This means fuel for our brain and muscles, rather than fat storage. Studies have shown that the consumption of coconut oil can assist in calorie burning, fat oxidation and reduced food intake, and as a result, weight loss.

Additional health benefits include:
- Improved insulin sensitivity (and therefore Type 2 Diabetes control);
- Enhanced digestion and the alleviation of digestive disorders such as irritable bowel syndrome;
- Immunity. Coconut oil consists of lauric, caprylic and capric acids all of which have fantastic antibacterial and antiviral properties.

What brand should I buy?

Look for an *unrefined organic extra virgin* coconut oil. Unrefined coconut oil undergoes less processing and retains its signature coconut flavour.

Extra virgin simply means fresh, raw coconut without the addition of any chemicals. Unfortunately there are no current industry standards in Australia for exactly what 'virgin' or 'extra virgin' means.

Coconut Revolution is by far the best there is. You can check out their entire product range here: www.coconutrevolution.com.au.

Please avoid coconut oil spray as we are not trying to limit our fat intake (oil sprays were originally invented in the low-fat era to minimise the amount used), and we do not need butane and propane in our food either.

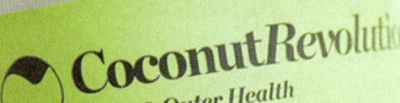

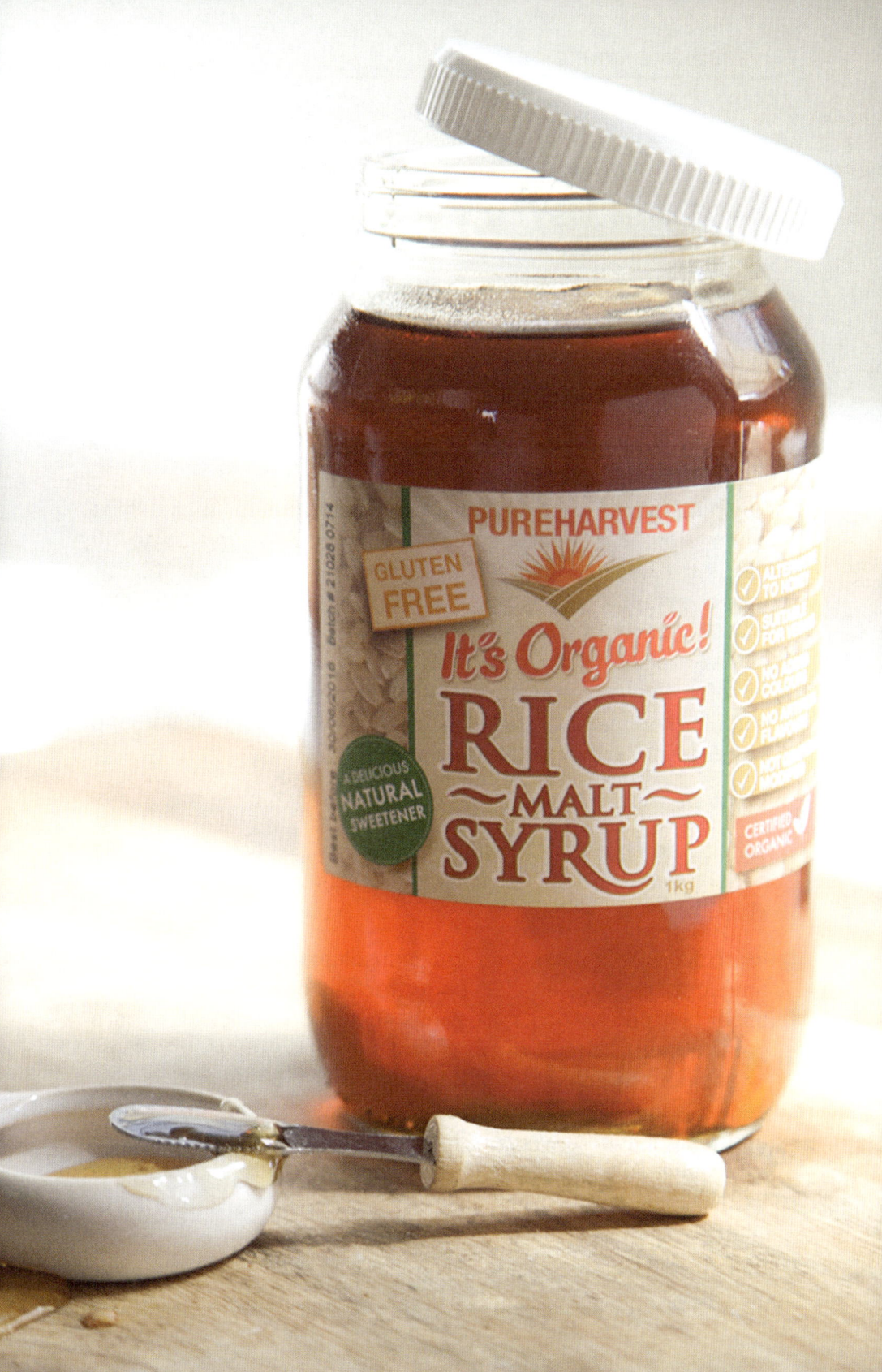

Rice malt syrup

Rice malt syrup is made from 100% organic brown rice. It is made through culturing rice with enzymes to breakdown the starches and then cooking until it becomes syrup. The final product contains soluble complex carbohydrates, maltose and a small amount of glucose. Rice malt syrup is 100% fructose free.

Why is fructose free important?

The importance here is that the carbohydrates in rice malt syrup provide a steady supply of energy, requiring up to 90 minutes digestion time. Other sweeteners like sugar, honey, maple syrup, coconut sugar and agave, which range from 50-90% fructose, are faster releasing sugars which cause insulin spikes, the associated blood sugar crashes and therefore cravings, hunger and fatigue. As we have discussed, chronically elevated insulin levels lead to fat accumulation and longer term, obesity and diabetes.

What are the other benefits of rice malt syrup?

Other than an efficient source of energy, rice malt syrup is the perfect sweetener for those following a low-fructose diet, and unlike honey, is suitable for vegans.

In cooking or baking, you can substitute rice malt syrup for any sugar or sweetener. Even for recipes requiring one cup of sugar, 1/4 cup of rice malt syrup should be sufficient. What's great about rice malt syrup is that unlike our more traditional sweeteners, it doesn't taste too sweet. This helps with portion control and again, blood sugar control, satiety, hormonal control and weight management. In case you hadn't noticed, sweet foods stimulate the need for more sweet foods and start the vicious cycle of addiction.

Why wouldn't you use rice malt syrup?

As it is made from brown rice, rice malt syrup is technically not grain free. Those following a strict Paleo protocol usually use honey or maple syrup as sweeteners for this reason, but please be mindful of the fructose content here.

Note: those following a low carbohydrate protocol should use rice malt syrup infrequently. It contains 8 grams of carbohydrate per 10 gram serve (80% carbohydrate) and the reason why sweet treats are exactly that: 'treats'.

What brand should I buy?

Pure Harvest. They are one of Australia's largest manufacturers and distributors of natural and organic food and pride themselves on unadulterated chemical-free products. Importantly, their rice malt syrup is GMO-free. You can purchase yours from the health food section of the supermarket. For more information visit www.pureharvest.com.au.

Quinoa

Quinoa, (pronounced keen-wa), is the seed of the Chenopodium or Goosefoot plant. It is gluten free, grain free, high protein and packed full of nutrients including calcium, iron, zinc and B vitamins. It is classed as a superfood and a good carbohydrate choice post training.

Quinoa is delicious as a porridge or bircher muesli, or as a grain free substitute to rice. It's also fantastic to bulk up salads, soups and casseroles.

Whilst it is grain free, some people experience digestive problems with quinoa. The seed coating contains saponins which can irritate the intestines, so quinoa must be soaked and washed under running water thoroughly before cooking.

Here is how to prepare quinoa:

1. Soak 1 cup of quinoa for 15 minutes then rinse under running water. You can tell when the saponin is removed, as it produces a soapy solution in the water.
2. Drain the quinoa and add to 2 cups of boiling water.
3. Bring to the boil, and then turn the heat down to simmer. Fluff gently with a fork mid-way. Cook for 20 minutes or until the edge of the seed separates as a white spiral and the seed turns clear. All of the water should have evaporated.
4. Remove from the heat and allow to sit for five minutes before serving.
5. Store in an airtight container and add to your breakfast and salads during the week.

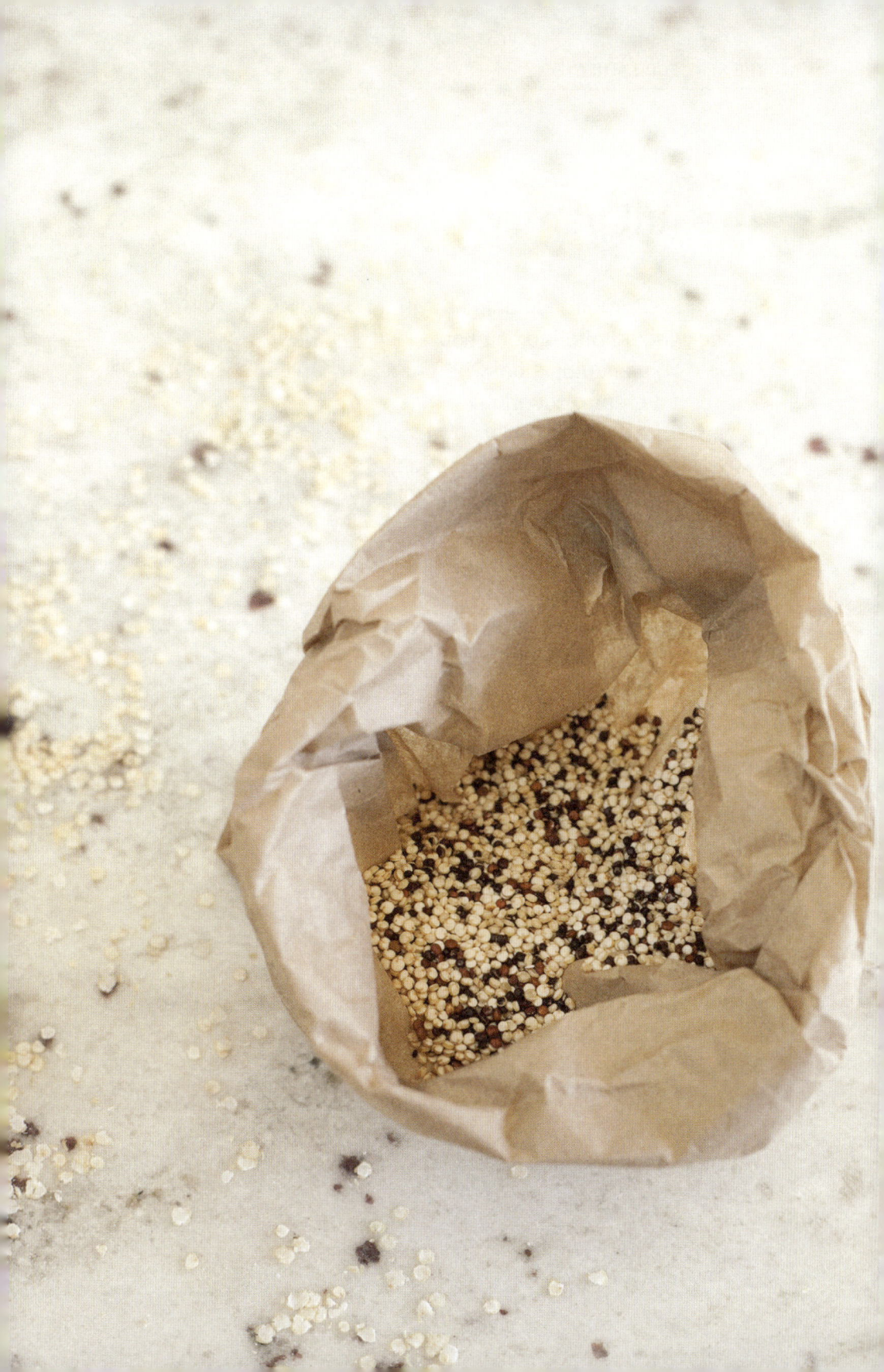

The full pantry

- Flours: almond meal, hazelnut meal, coconut flour, buckwheat flour, tapioca flour
- Dairy substitutes: unsweetened nut milk, coconut milk, coconut cream, coconut yoghurt
- Nuts: almonds, hazelnuts, macadamias, cashews, walnuts
- Seeds: pepitas, sunflower seeds, chia seeds, tahini
- Fats: coconut oil, macadamia oil, olive oil, nut butters, grass-fed butter
- Cacao and coconut: cacao powder, cacao nibs, coconut flakes, shredded coconut
- Natural sweetness: rice malt syrup, Medjool dates, Natvia
- Quinoa: quinoa seeds, quinoa flakes
- Spices: cinnamon, nutmeg, turmeric, chilli flakes, mixed Italian herbs
- Gluten free baking powder
- Sea salt
- Eggs
- Apple cider vinegar

Ingredients

Most ingredients are available from any health food store or in the health food aisle of your local supermarket. The most economical way though, is to buy in bulk. To save on cost, why not order with a friend or two. A fantastic online shop is: Bulk Whole Foods Australia (www.thenaturalnutritionist.com.au/BWF).

Your list is available as a standalone shopping list on the next page.

Shopping list

Flours	Nuts	Fats	Natural Sweetness	Spices
Almond meal	Almonds	Coconut oil	Rice malt syrup	Cinnamon
Hazelnut meal	Hazelnuts	Macadamia oil	Medjool dates	Nutmeg
Coconut flour	Macadamias	Olive oil	Natvia	Turmeric
Buckwheat flour	Cashews	Nut butter e.g. almond, cashew		Chilli flakes
Tapioca flour	Walnuts	Grass-fed butter		Mixed herbs

Dairy Substitutes	Seeds	Cacao and Coconut	Quinoa	Other
Unsweetened nut milk	Pepitas	Cacao powder	Quinoa seeds	Gluten free baking powder
Coconut milk	Sunflower seeds	Cacao nibs	Quinoa flakes	Sea salt
Coconut cream	Chia seeds	Coconut flakes		Eggs
Coconut yoghurt	Tahini	Shredded coconut		Apple cider vinegar

Gut Health 101

As we discussed in Part 1, gut health is incredibly important, as your gut is your second brain. The best place to start is where you are comfortable, and here are a number of options to start your gut health journey. Please note: it is not a matter of 'more is more' as you can over-do even the good bacteria. Please start gradually and build your intake over the next four weeks.

Fermented vegetables

Fermented vegetables are one of the easiest and most convenient sources of good bacteria. Fermented foods in general contain millions of beneficial microbes, which drive out pathogens and therefore protect gut integrity. In addition, the bacteria pre-digest our food, which means we have greater access to nutrients. There is actually 20 times more bioavailable vitamin C in sauerkraut than in fresh cabbage.

Fermented vegetables are also the most economical place to start. To make sauerkraut, finely shred one cabbage and transfer into a large bowl. Add one tablespoon of quality salt and use your hands to squeeze as much juice out of the cabbage as possible. If you're patient, you should get enough liquid so that when transferred into an airtight container, it is completely covered. For large cabbages, you may like to split this process into two. Salt is essential to create the right environment (pH) for fermentation to take place.

From here, all you need to do it store your well-packed cabbage on the kitchen bench for 4-7 days. From there, transfer into the fridge and enjoy. You can actually use any vegetables you like (for example, carrots, beetroot, daikon, and artichokes), in any combination, and add any herbs and spices you desire. Serve 1-2 tablespoons on your eggs, in a salad, or as a side to any main meal.

If you prefer to purchase your fermented vegetables, Peace, Love and Vegetables (www.peaceloveandvegetables.com.au) is available in the fridge section of most health food stores.

Bone broth

Bone broth is one of nature's true superfoods. It is packed full of calcium, magnesium and phosphorus and provides gelatin and collagen for cell integrity and healing. While everyone will benefit from adding bone broth, it is absolutely essential for those with leaky gut, celiac disease, Hashimoto's and other autoimmune conditions.

This mineral rich drink or stock is also one of the best ways to ensure your kitchen is wastage free. Your Super Easy Bone Broth recipe (page 214) is a great place to start.

If you are not quite ready to make your own, you can buy online at Broth of Life (www.brothoflife.com.au) and rehydrate as required.

Yoghurt

A probiotic yoghurt is one of the simplest was to regularly consume fermented foods. Kultured Wellness have created a fantastic starter culture that needs to be become your predominate gut health food.

Here's why:
- It's fermentation made easy. All you need to do is purchase your starter culture and add to coconut cream to make yoghurt or coconut water to make kefir. No elaborate equipment and only a small investment of time.
- They contain ten strains of good bacteria, which is important for microbiome diversity. Many probiotics contain only two strains.
- They are extremely high potency. It's one cup per day or an entire bottle of probiotics.
- The cultures are D-Lactate free to benefit people with issues such as MTHFR, and liver and detox problems.
- They contain high numbers of Bifidobacterium, which are important for leaky gut, immune regulation and digesting plant matter.
- They are vegan-friendly, free from additives, preservatives or fillers.
- One starter can be used to make approximately 10 litres of kefir or yoghurt. That's $4/L and one of the most cost effective ways to prioritise your gut health.

To get started purchase your starter culture online at www.thenaturalnutritionist.com.au/kultured-wellness and see page 216 for detailed instructions.

Kefir

Kefir is a probiotic drink made from 'grains' (tibicos), which act like the starter culture in yoghurt. Traditionally the grains are added to milk and fermented via the lactose, or milk sugar. For a dairy free and vegan option, we can again turn to Kultured Wellness. Full instructions can be found on page 216, but it is as simple as combining with coconut water in a glass jar and fermenting on the bench for 4-7 days. Check out our Fermented Chia Pudding on page 224 for a delicious and nutrient dense way to strengthen your gut health.

If you're not quite ready to DIY, Peace, Love and Vegetables make a fantastic coconut kefir is dairy free, sugar free, delicious and available in health food stores.

Kombucha

Kombucha is made from a starter culture (known as a Symbiotic Colony Of Bacteria and Yeast or "SCOBY"), sugar and tea. When double fermented, it becomes a fruity fizzy drink and a great replacement for soft drink, as hard as it may be to believe.

To make your own, obtain a SCOBY from someone already brewing their own kombucha tea, purchase one from a reputable source or grow one from a bottle of raw (i.e. unpasteurized) kombucha tea. Cultures for Health (www.culturesforhealth.com) is a fantastic online resource.

If you're not ready to make your own Remedy Kombucha is available from the fridge section of most health food stores. For more information please visit www.remedykombucha.com.au.

For more gut-loving eats, head to page 224.

Eating out

Eating out is simple once you are proficient with 2/1/2. Most restaurants offer gluten free and/or Paleo options, and there are many real food cafes popping up all over the world. Make your cafe or restaurant choice wisely and there will be plenty of options for you to select from the menu.

The best cuisines to start with are:
1. Japanese
2. Greek
3. Spanish
4. Thai
5. Indian

All are relatively easy to navigate (think meats, vegetables, curries and broths), but please consider that many sauces, including soy, contain gluten. Additionally, chips or fries often contain wheat, so please be mindful of this if you are treating yourself. Opt for hand-cut chips and fill your plate with vegetables, quality protein and good fats so you are less likely to over-consume. A failsafe method is to always request gluten free when ordering.

When choosing Thai, Indian or Japanese, simply double the vegetables and protein and control your portion of rice (or skip it altogether). If you do consume rice, order coconut rice where possible as the extra fat will reduce your blood sugar response.

Alternatively, here are some simple options to get you started:

- Eggs, bacon, spinach, tomato, mushrooms and avocado
- An omelette with a side of avocado
- Calamari salad with avocado
- Chicken and roast vegetable salad - check the dressing is olive oil based
- Steak and salad or vegetables - ask which sauce is gluten free or request butter instead
- Grilled fish or salmon and salad, with sweet potato fries if available
- Prawn served with Greek salad
- Open gyros - ask for no bread and extra fillings
- Kokoretsi (seasoned lamb innards baked until crispy) with horta (boiled greens served with lemon and olive oil)
- A chilli, garlic and ginger stir fry - ask for extra vegetables instead of rice
- Thai coconut and vegetable broth
- Green chicken curry - ask for extra vegetables and serve with half a cup of coconut rice
- Sashimi and seaweed salad
- Chicken yakitori and shitake mushrooms
- Asian chicken salad
- San choi bau
- Pho - sub noodles for extra vegetables
- Goi ga (chicken and cabbage salad)
- Vietnamese beef salad
- Whole fish with Vietnamese salad

Travelling

These days, most restaurants are providing fantastic real food options but unfortunately the same can't be said for airports and aeroplanes. The solution? BYO.

Here are some great combinations to pack, depending on the duration of the flight.

Short flight (1-3 hours): A large meal prior such as a Three-Egg Omelette, with a small portion of nuts as a back up.

Medium flight (3-5 hours): Pack a glass container with spinach, avocado, tomato, capsicum and feta and take protein in the form of a can of sardines, smoked salmon or boiled eggs to add. People may complain about the smell of fish on a plane but the inflight meals can smell far worse! Great snacks are Coconut and Raspberry Delights, Chocolate Brownie Bites, chopped carrot sticks and hummus, a punnet of berries or a portable container of nuts.

Long flight (5+ hours): Make sure you're well fed before a long haul and take as much of the above as possible. The best thing about natural whole foods and monitoring your carbohydrate intake is that you just won't have the same insatiable hunger, so travelling becomes far less stressful from a fuelling point of view. Keep this in mind on a day-to-day basis too – they key is satiety after all, so if you are hungry within four hours, start by adding more fats followed by non-starchy vegetables to your meals.

If you haven't pre-prepared then pick up a salad with good fats, vegetables and protein from Sumo Salad or Subway, but it's never going to be anywhere near as tasty or nutritious as something you have made yourself. The more you travel, the more organised you will become.

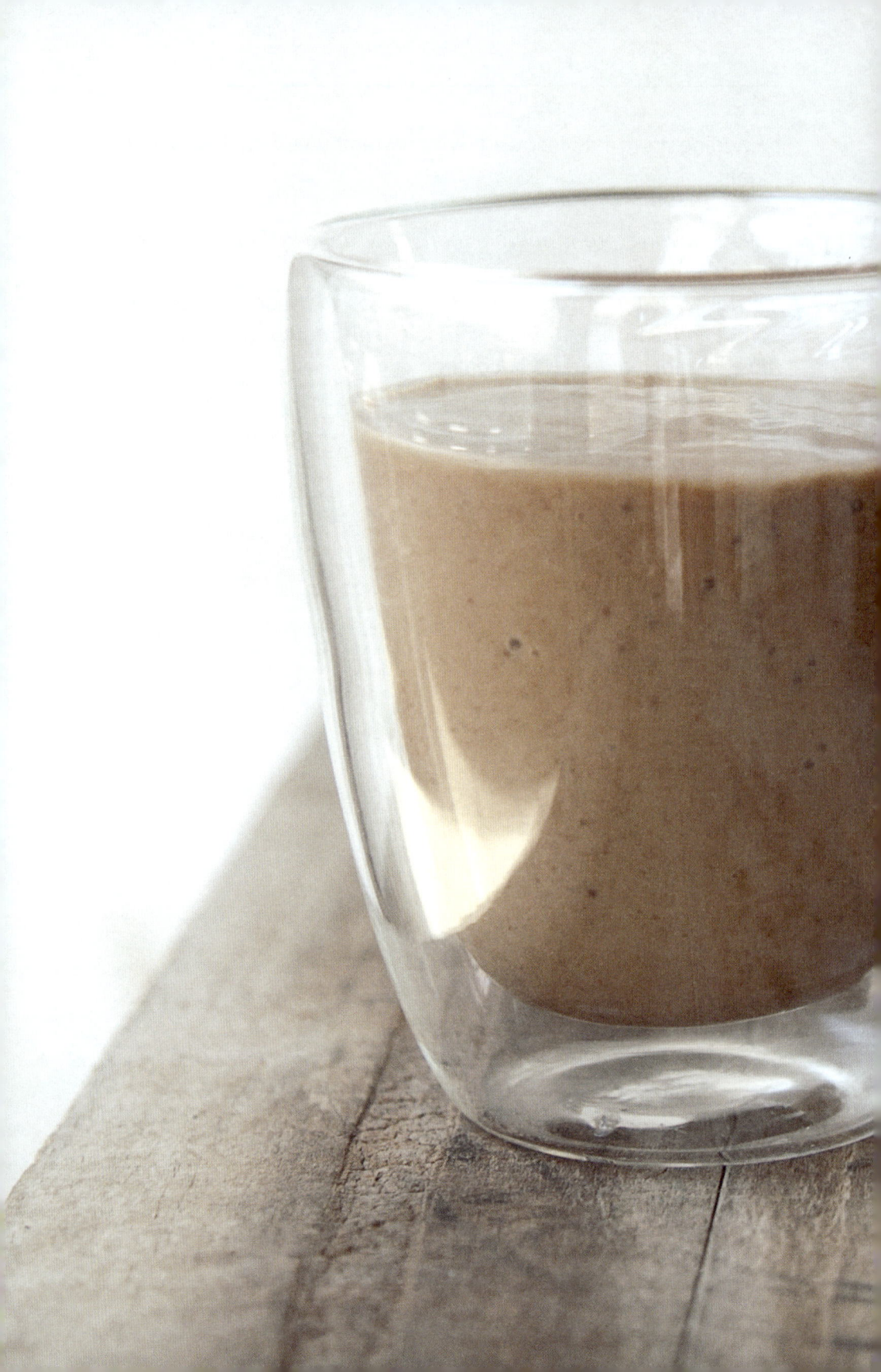

PART 4
RECIPES

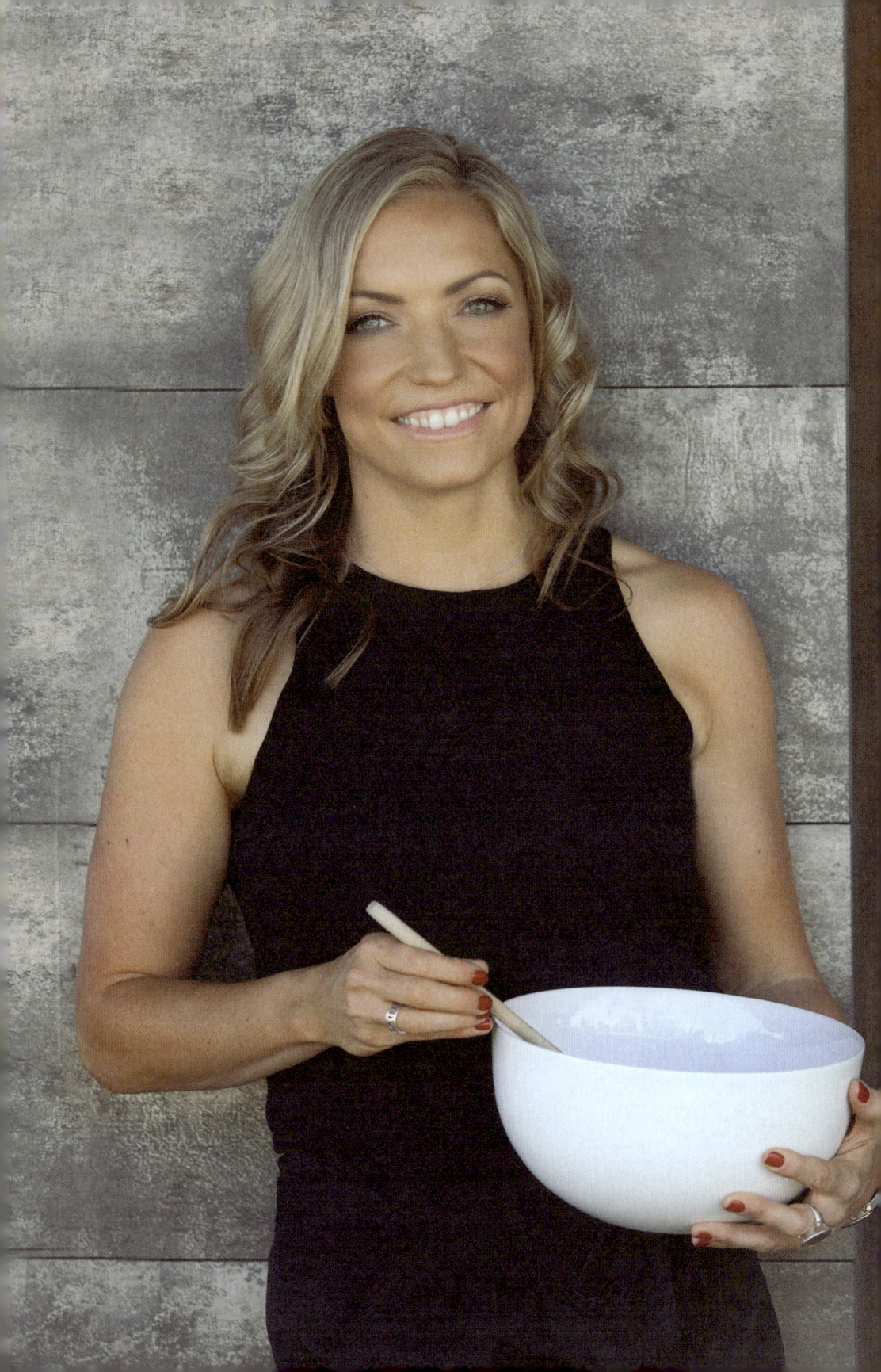

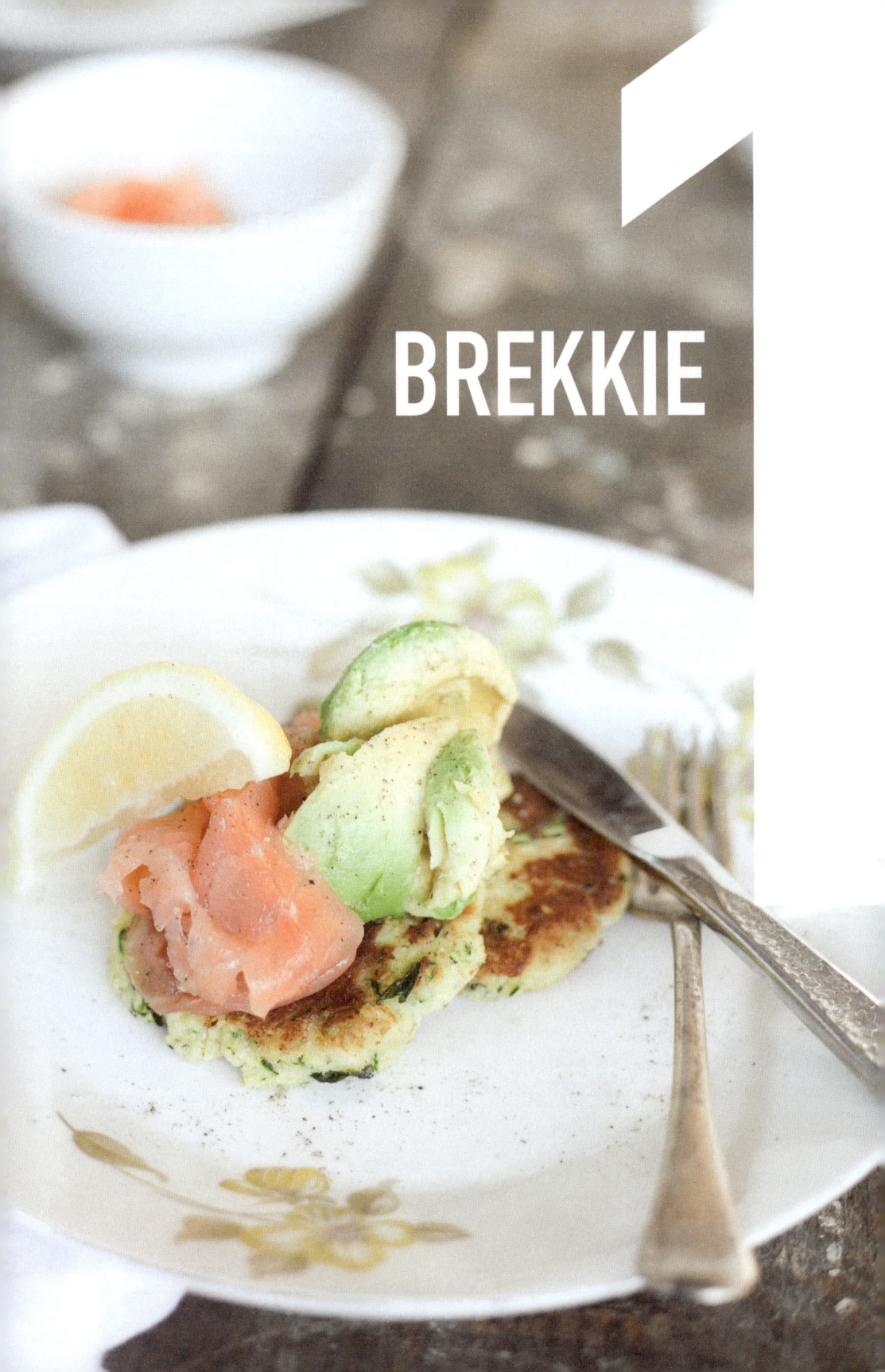

BREKKIE 1

Breakfast Antioxidant Smoothie

Ingredients (Serves 1)
- 1 cup water
- 1 teaspoon chia seeds
- 1/4 cup coconut cream
- 1/2 avocado
- 1 tablespoon cashew butter
- 1 handful spinach
- 1 handful cos lettuce
- 1/4 cup raspberries
- 1 teaspoon cinnamon
- 1 tablespoon cold-pressed extra virgin coconut oil
- 1 scoop quality protein powder, such as Bare Blends
- 1/3 -1 tray ice

Toppings:
- 1 handful walnuts, crushed
- Cacao nibs, to taste

Method
1. Add water and chia seeds to the blender and let sit for 15 minutes for the chia seeds to go to work.
2. Add cream, avo, cashew butter, spinach, cos, raspberries, cinnamon, and oil and blend well.
3. Add protein powder and ice and blend until thick but smooth. Add more ice for a thicker smoothie.
4. Pour into a bowl, add toppings and enjoy. Easily transported in a jar if required.

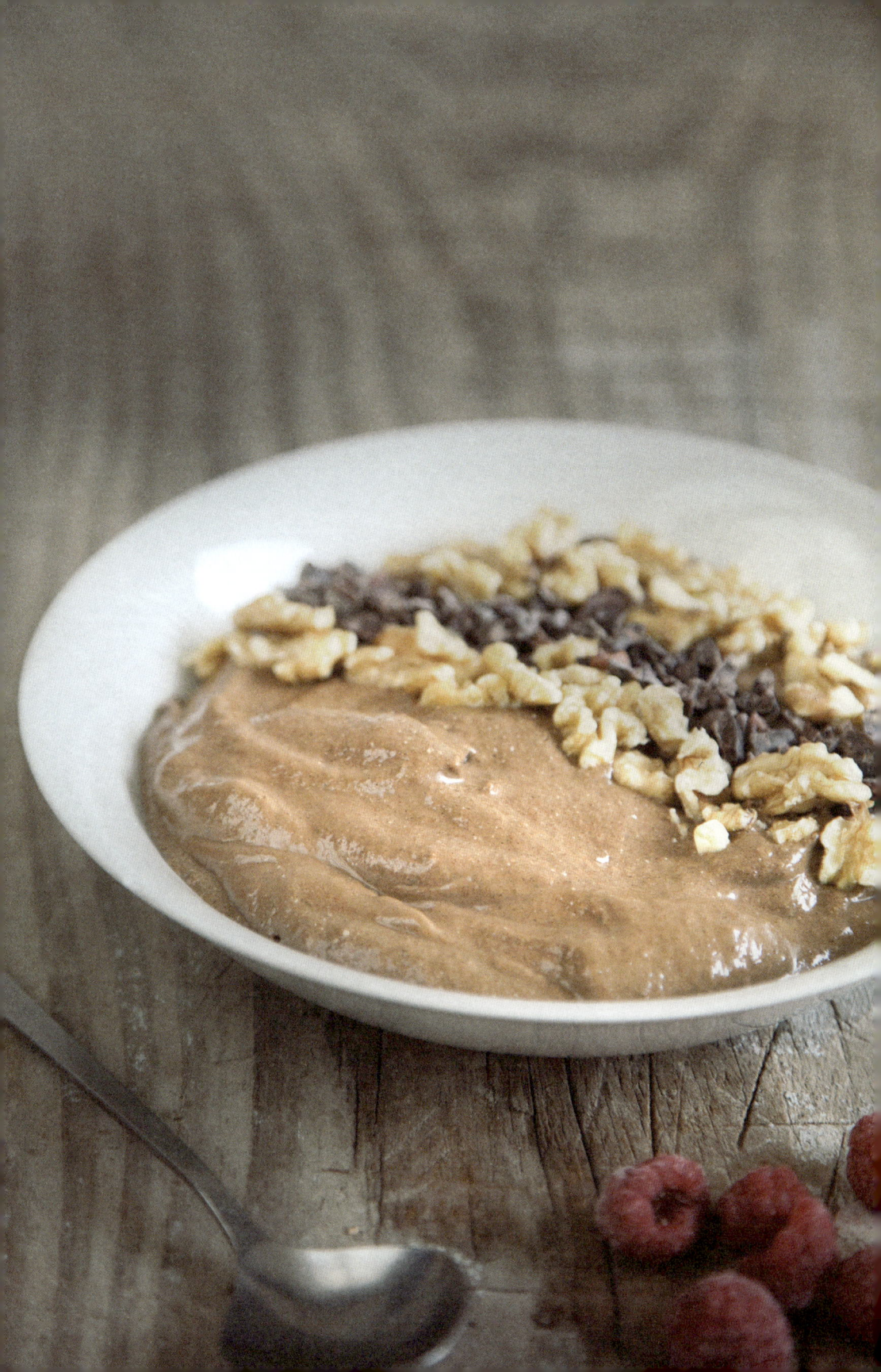

Chocolate Avocado Smoothie

Ingredients (Serves 1)
- 1/2 cup unsweetened almond milk
- 1/2 avocado
- 1 Medjool date, pitted
- 1 teaspoon raw cacao nibs
- 1 teaspoon cinnamon
- 1 teaspoon chia seeds
- 1 large handful spinach
- 1 scoop quality protein powder, such as Bare Blends
- 1 tray of ice

Method
1. Combine all the ingredients in a blender and blend until smooth.
2. Top with extra cacao nibs and enjoy.

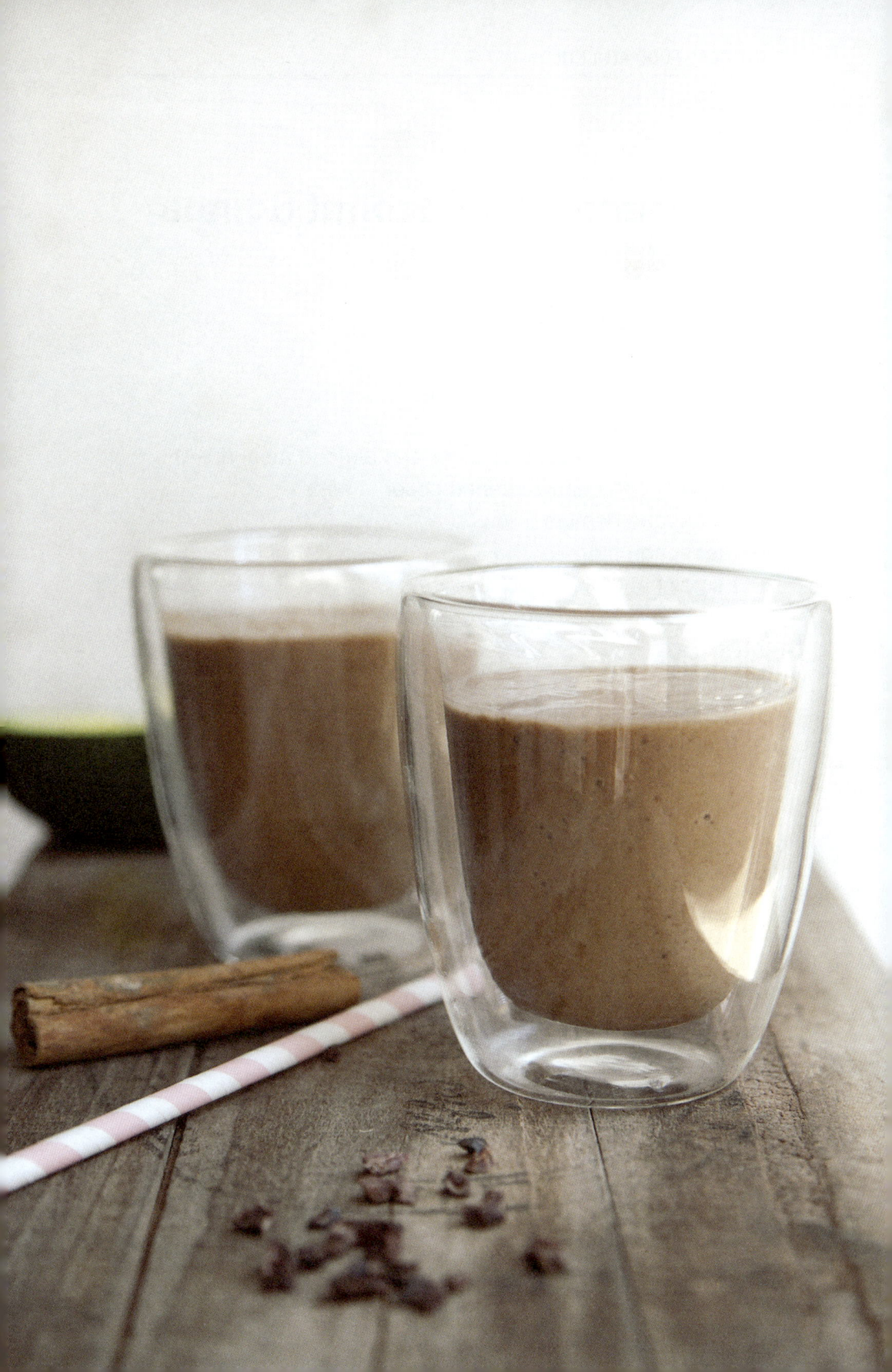

Raspberry and Coconut Quinoa Porridge

Ingredients (Serves 1)
- 1/2 cup water
- 1 cup unsweetened nut milk
- 1/2 cup quinoa flakes
- 1 teaspoon linseed, sunflower and almond meal (LSA)
- 2 tablespoons unsweetened coconut flakes
- 1 teaspoon pepitas
- 1 teaspoon nutmeg
- 1 small handful raspberries
- 1 teaspoon Pure Harvest organic rice malt syrup

Method
1. Bring water and half of the milk to the boil.
2. Add quinoa and cook for 2-3 minutes, stirring well until thick and all the liquid has evaporated.
3. Pour into a bowl and stir through LSA.
4. Top with coconut, pepitas, remaining milk and nutmeg.
5. Add raspberries and drizzle rice malt syrup on top.

Other great toppings to try:
- Cashew, banana and date.
- Chopped banana and walnuts.
- A handful of blueberries.
- Grated apple and almonds.

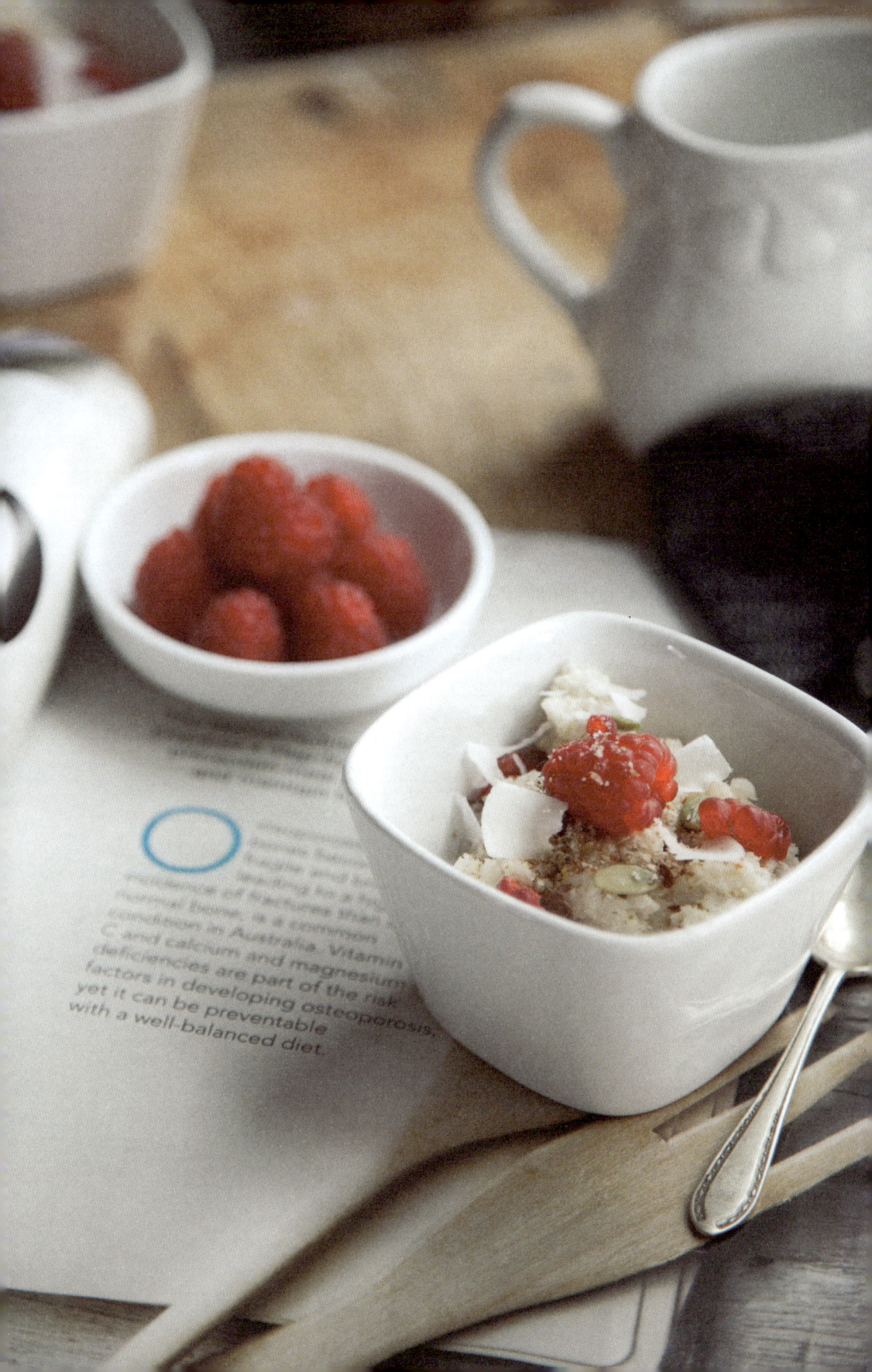

Sugar Free Breakfast Cereal

Ingredients (Serves 1)
- 2 tablespoons unsweetened coconut flakes
- 2 teaspoons pepitas
- 8 walnuts halves, crushed
- 1 teaspoon chia seeds
- 150g Greek/coconut yogurt
- 1 small handful of raspberries

Method
1. Combine coconut, pepitas, walnuts and chia seeds in a small bowl.
2. Add yoghurt and berries and stir thoroughly. Pop in the fridge for a few minutes to allow the chia seeds to expand and form a delicious parfait.

Short on time in the morning? Why not make up containers of the nuts and seeds as part of your Sunday food prep, that way you only need to add yogurt and berries and your breakfast will be ready in one minute flat.

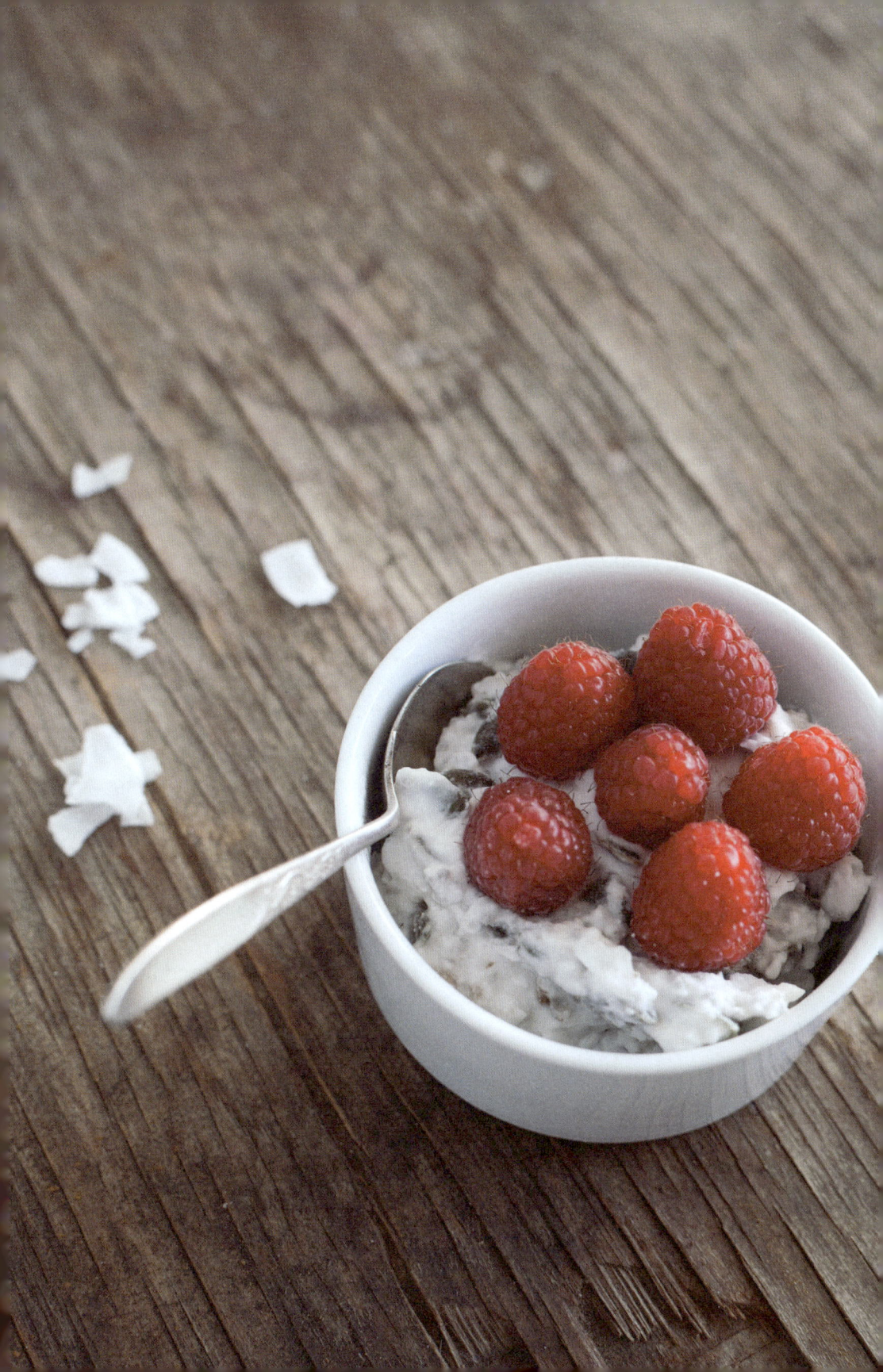

Coconut, Raspberry and Cacao Chia Pudding

Ingredients (Serves 1)

Pudding:
- 3 tablespoons chia seeds
- 1 cup unsweetened almond milk
- 1 teaspoon Pure Harvest organic rice malt syrup
- 1 teaspoon pure vanilla extract
- 1/4 cup raspberries
- 8 almonds, chopped

Toppings:
- A couple of raspberries
- 1 small handful cacao nibs
- 1 small handful unsweetened coconut flakes
- A drizzle of rice malt syrup, optional

Method
1. Combine all pudding ingredients in an airtight container, stir thoroughly and soak overnight in the fridge. You may need to check on it once or twice and stir again.
2. Serve with raspberries, cacao nibs, coconut flakes and if you need a little more sweetness, rice malt syrup.

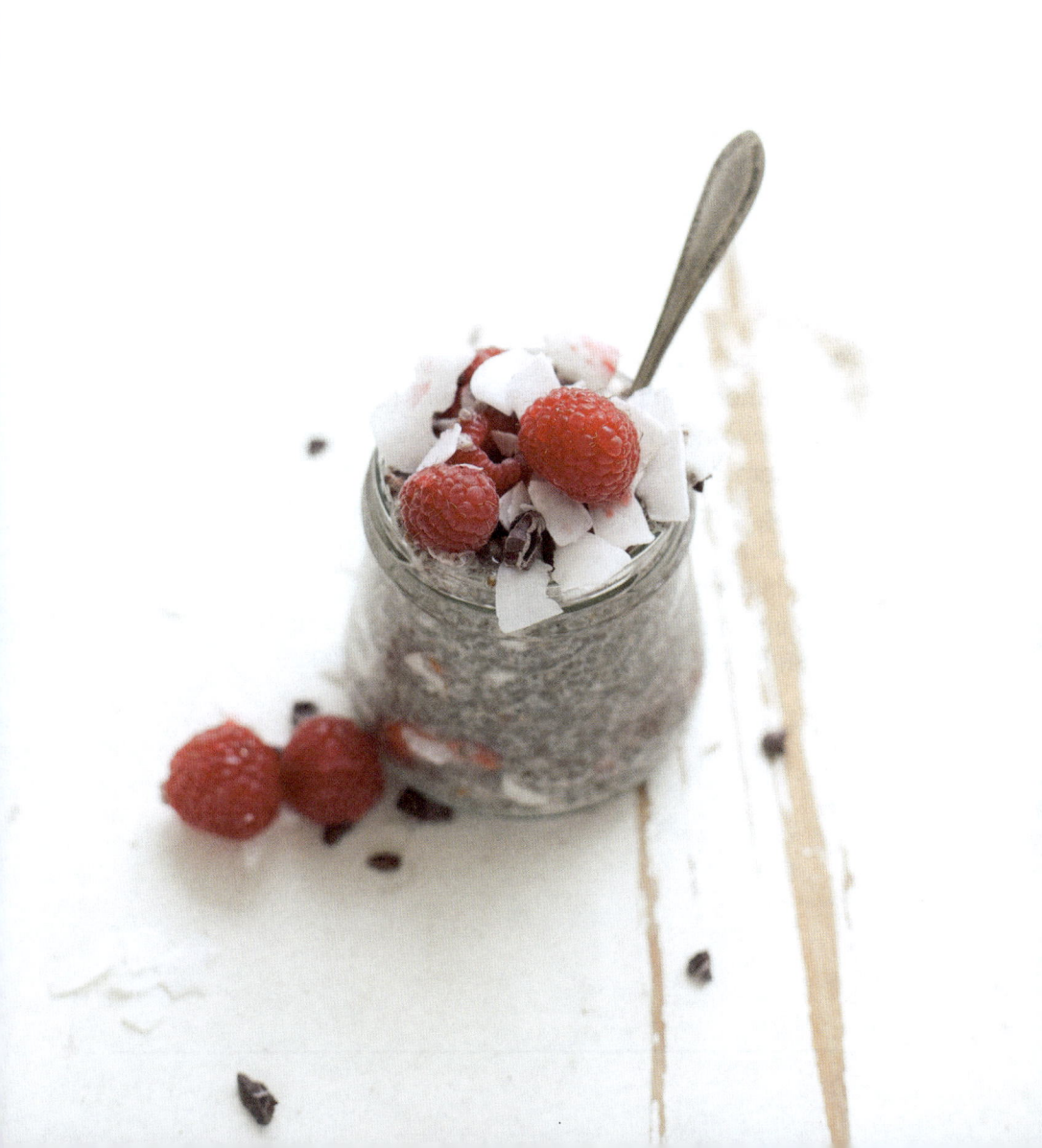

All Natural Low Carb Gluten Free Bread

Ingredients (Makes 10-12 slices)
- 1 1/2 cups almond flour
- 1/4 cup coconut flour
- 1/4 cup linseed, sunflower and almond meal (LSA)
- 1/4 teaspoon sea salt
- 2 teaspoons gluten free baking powder
- 5 eggs, free range
- 1/4 cup cold-pressed extra virgin coconut oil
- 1 tablespoon Pure Harvest organic rice malt syrup
- 1 tablespoon apple cider vinegar (ACV)

Method
1. Preheat oven to 180°C.
2. Blend almond flour, coconut flour, LSA, salt and baking powder together. Pour into a large bowl.
3. In a separate bowl, beat eggs.
4. Add the eggs, oil, rice malt syrup and ACV and mix throughout.
5. Let sit until the liquid absorbs.
6. Scoop into a greased bread tin and bake for 30 minutes.
7. Cool and slice into 12 serves.

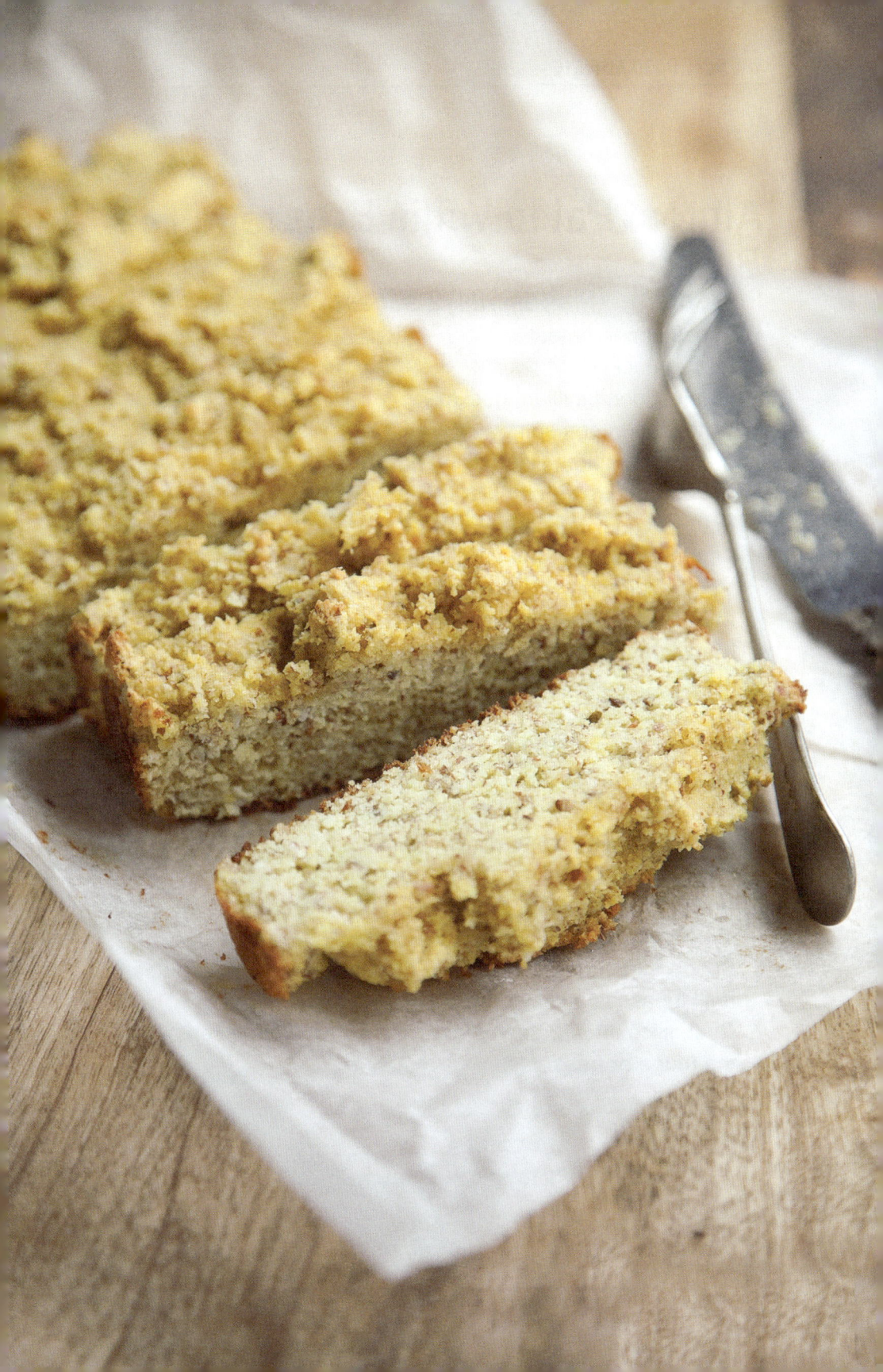

Almost Paleo Vegie Bread

Ingredients (Makes 10-12 slices)
- 2 cups almond meal
- 1/2 cup buckwheat flour
- 1 tablespoon psyllium husks
- 1/4 teaspoon sea salt
- 1 teaspoon gluten free baking powder
- 1 cup grated raw pumpkin
- 1 cup zucchini, grated
- 4 eggs, free range
- 1/4 cup cold-pressed extra virgin coconut oil, melted
- 1 tablespoon Pure Harvest organic rice malt syrup
- 1 tablespoon apple cider vinegar (ACV)

Method
1. Preheat oven to 180°C.
2. In a large bowl, combine almond meal, flour, psyllium, salt and baking powder.
3. Add grated vegetables to the bowl.
4. In a separate bowl, beat eggs.
5. Add the eggs, oil, rice malt syrup and ACV and mix thoroughly.
6. Scoop into a greased bread tin and bake for 30 minutes or until it passes a skewer test.
7. Cool, slice into 12 serves and store in an airtight container in the fridge or freezer.

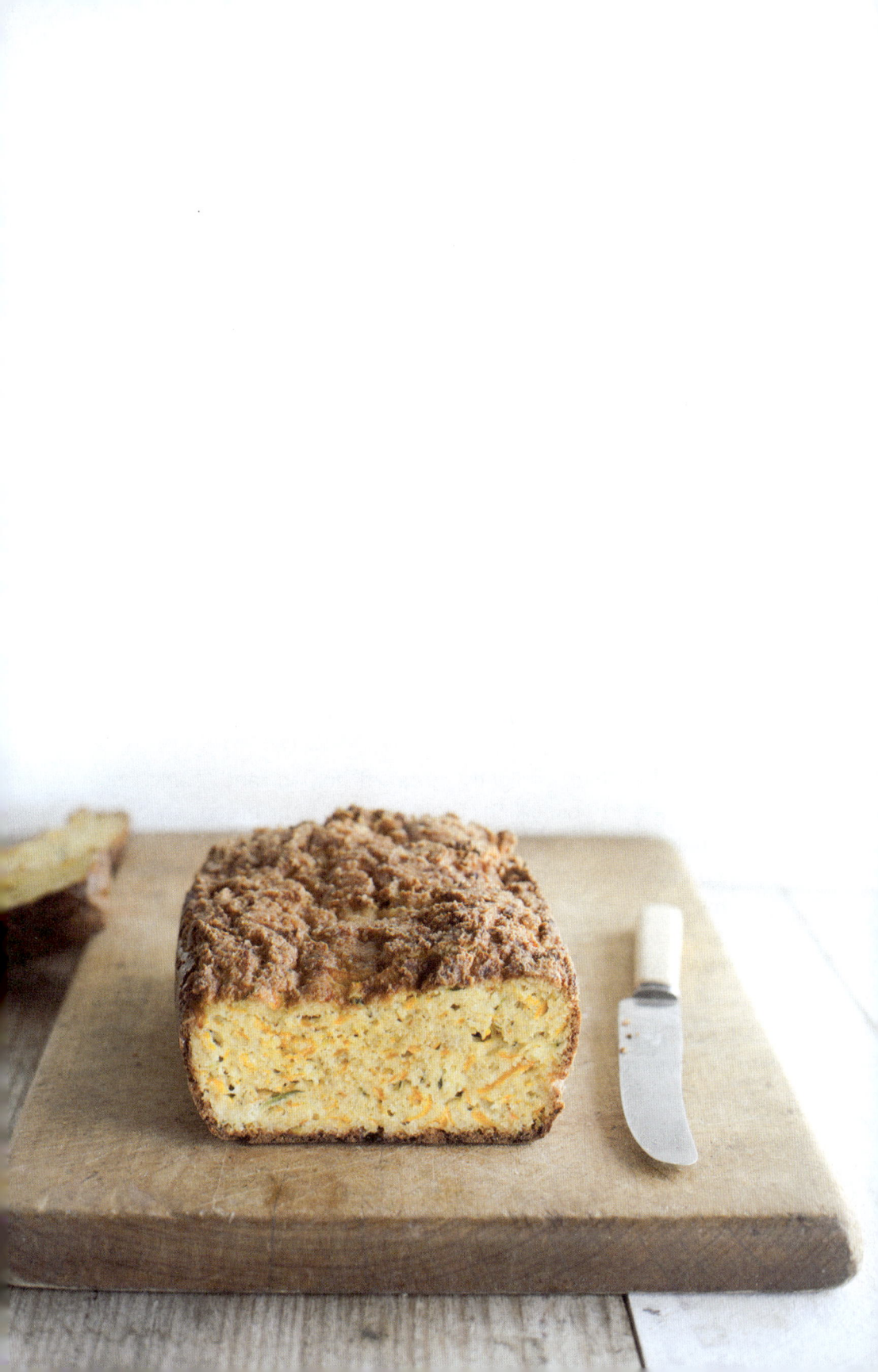

Three-Egg Omelette

Ingredients (Serves 1)
- 3 eggs, free range
- A dash of unsweetened coconut or almond milk
- 1 handful tomato, diced
- 1 small mushroom, diced
- 1 handful spinach, finely chopped
- 20g goat's feta (optional)
- Cold-pressed extra virgin coconut oil
- 2 slices All Natural Low Carb Gluten Free bread
- 1/2 avocado
- Sea salt and pepper, to taste

Method
1. Beat eggs and combine milk, tomato, mushroom and spinach in a large bowl.
2. Pour mix into a lightly greased frypan and cook until eggs are to your liking. Start to toast your bread while the omelette is cooking.
3. Sprinkle feta on one half of the omelette and gently fold in half.
4. Serve with toasted bread and avocado. Season with salt and pepper if desired.

Other great fillings to try:
- Leftover roasted vegies and sautéed onion.
- Mushroom, asparagus, pine nut and goat's feta.

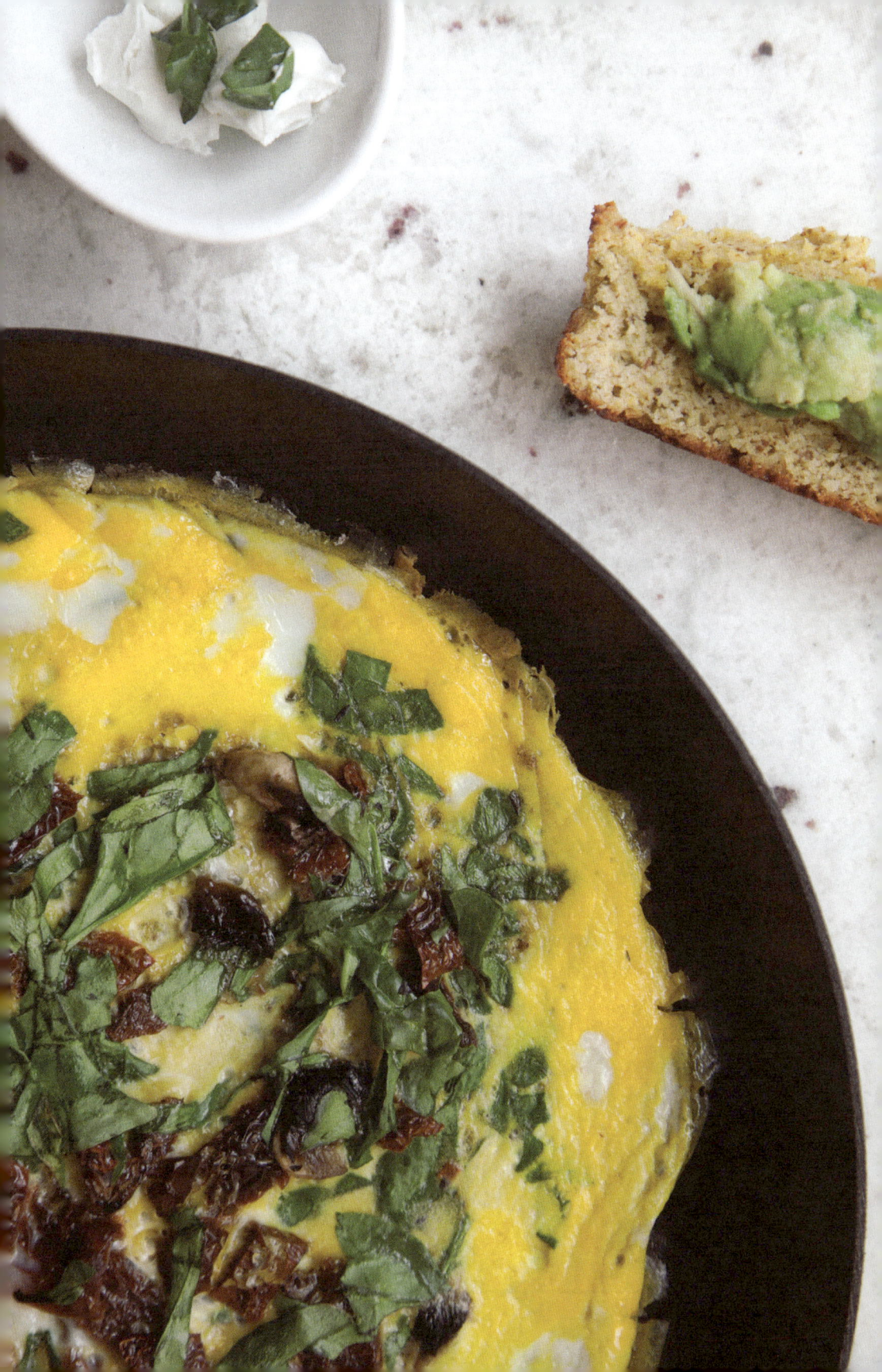

Breakfast Frittata

Ingredients (Serves 4)
- 8 eggs, free range
- 1/4 cup coconut cream
- 1 zucchini, grated
- 1/2 cup grated sweet potato
- 2 rashers bacon
- 1 teaspoon cold-pressed extra virgin coconut oil
- 1 tablespoon chilli flakes
- 1/4 teaspoon sea salt
- 1/4 teaspoon black pepper

Method
1. Preheat oven to 180°C.
2. Whisk eggs and coconut cream in a large bowl.
3. Add grated vegies.
4. Finely chop bacon and fry off in coconut oil. Add to the bowl with all other ingredients and combine well.
5. Pour into a round 20cm baking tin and cook for 20 minutes or until cooked through and firm to touch. Allow to cool slightly before slicing into quarters. Store leftovers in the fridge for 4-5 days.

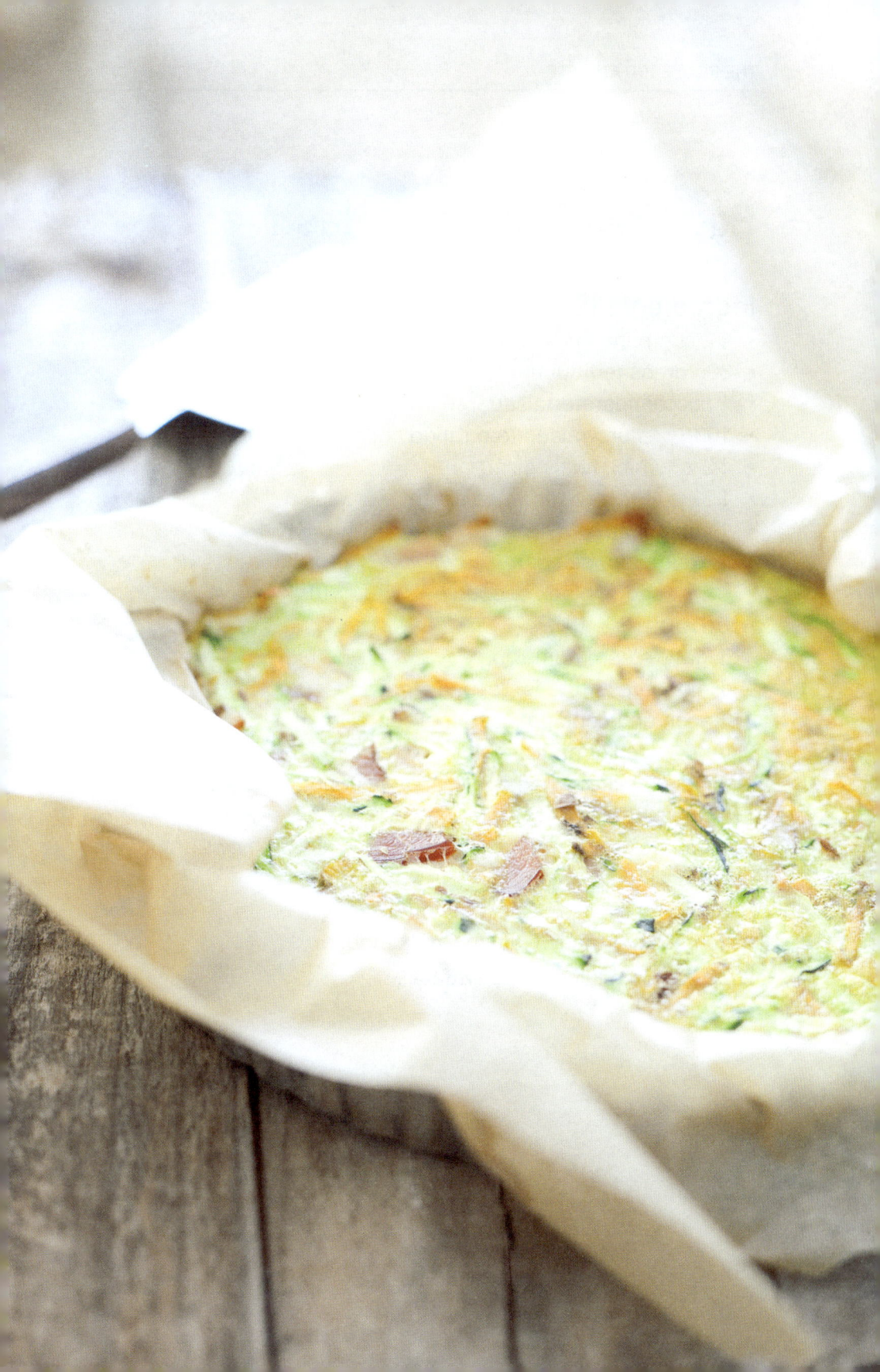

Egg Free Breakfast Hash

Ingredients (Serves 1)
- 1/2 cup pumpkin, chopped
- 30g grass-fed butter
- 1 rasher pasture-raised free range bacon, finely diced*
- 100g pasture-raised free range chorizo, finely diced*
- 1/2 zucchini, finely diced
- 1/2 cup broccoli, floretted small
- 1 cup spinach
- 1/2 avocado, diced

Method
1. Lightly steam pumpkin.
2. Heat butter in a large pan and add pumpkin, chorizo and bacon and cook until caramelised, stirring throughout.
3. Add zucchini and broccoli and cook for one to two minutes or until well covered and slightly softened.
4. Add spinach and stir through well.
5. Remove from the heat, transfer into a bowl, top with avocado and enjoy.

*A fantastic brand is Gamze Smokehouse: www.gamzesmokehouse.com.au.

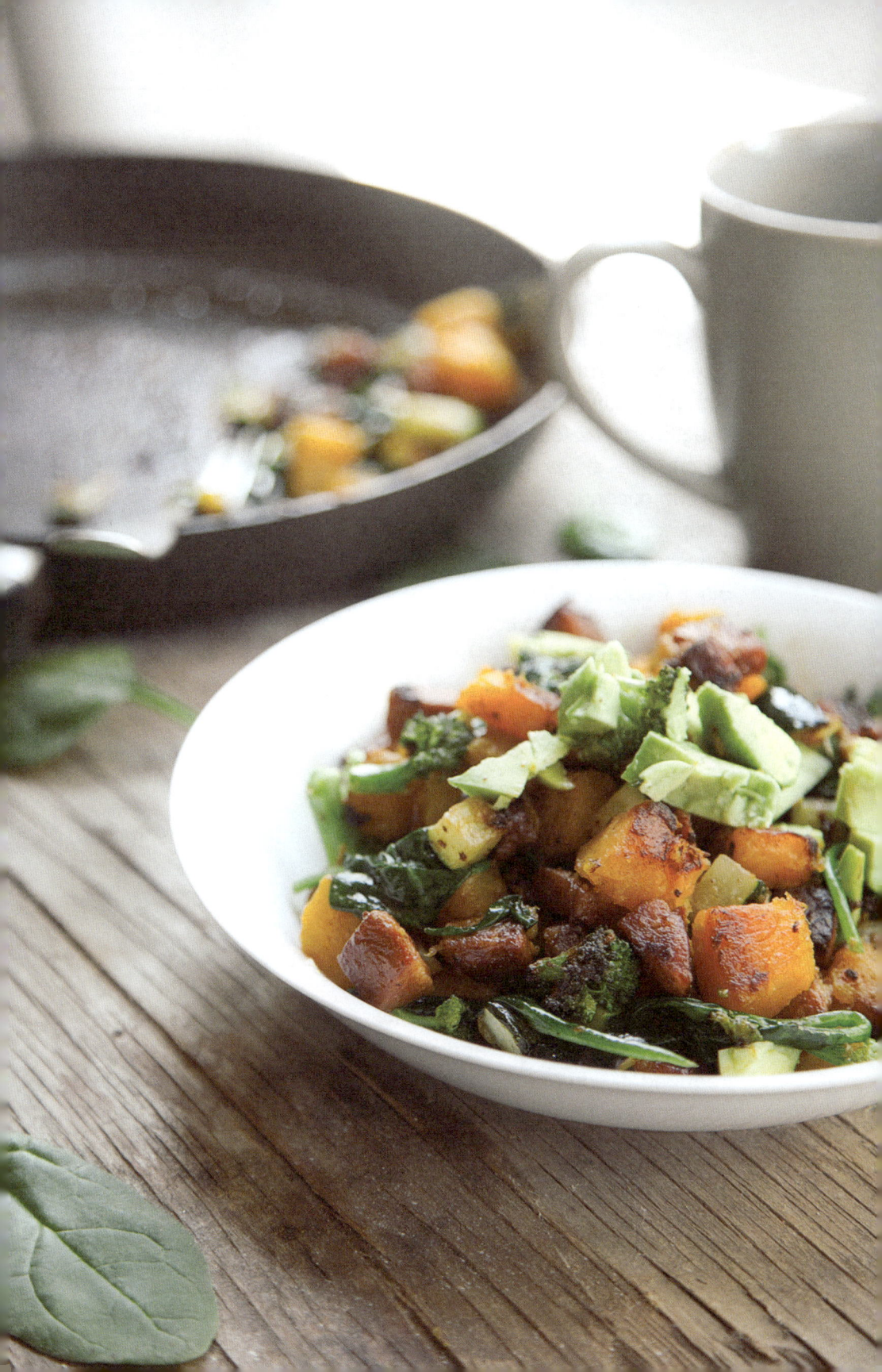

Zucchini, Mint and Feta Fritters

Ingredients (Makes 6 fritters)
Fritters:
- 2 eggs, free range
- 1 zucchini, grated
- 1 large handful mint, finely chopped
- The juice of 1/2 lemon
- 1/4 cup goat's feta, crumbled
- 1/4 cup coconut flour, sifted
- 2 tablespoon psyllium
- A dash of water
- Black Pepper, to taste
- Cold-pressed extra virgin coconut oil, for frying

Toppings (per person):
- 2 slices smoked salmon
- 1/4 avocado, mashed
- 1 lemon wedge

Method
1. Whisk the eggs in a large bowl and add zucchini, mint, lemon and feta.
2. Add coconut flour and psyllium combine well. Add the water only if your mixture needs help binding.
3. Form medium balls, molding each well with your hands.
4. Heat coconut oil in a large frypan, flatten the fritters and fry two at a time, flipping half way with an egg-flip. Repeat for additional fritters, adding a touch more coconut oil if required. If you are just serving one, you can store the batter in the fridge and fry fresh the next day.
5. Serve two fritters topped with smoked salmon, avocado, fresh lemon and a sprinkle of black pepper. Any leftovers will keep for a couple of days in the fridge.

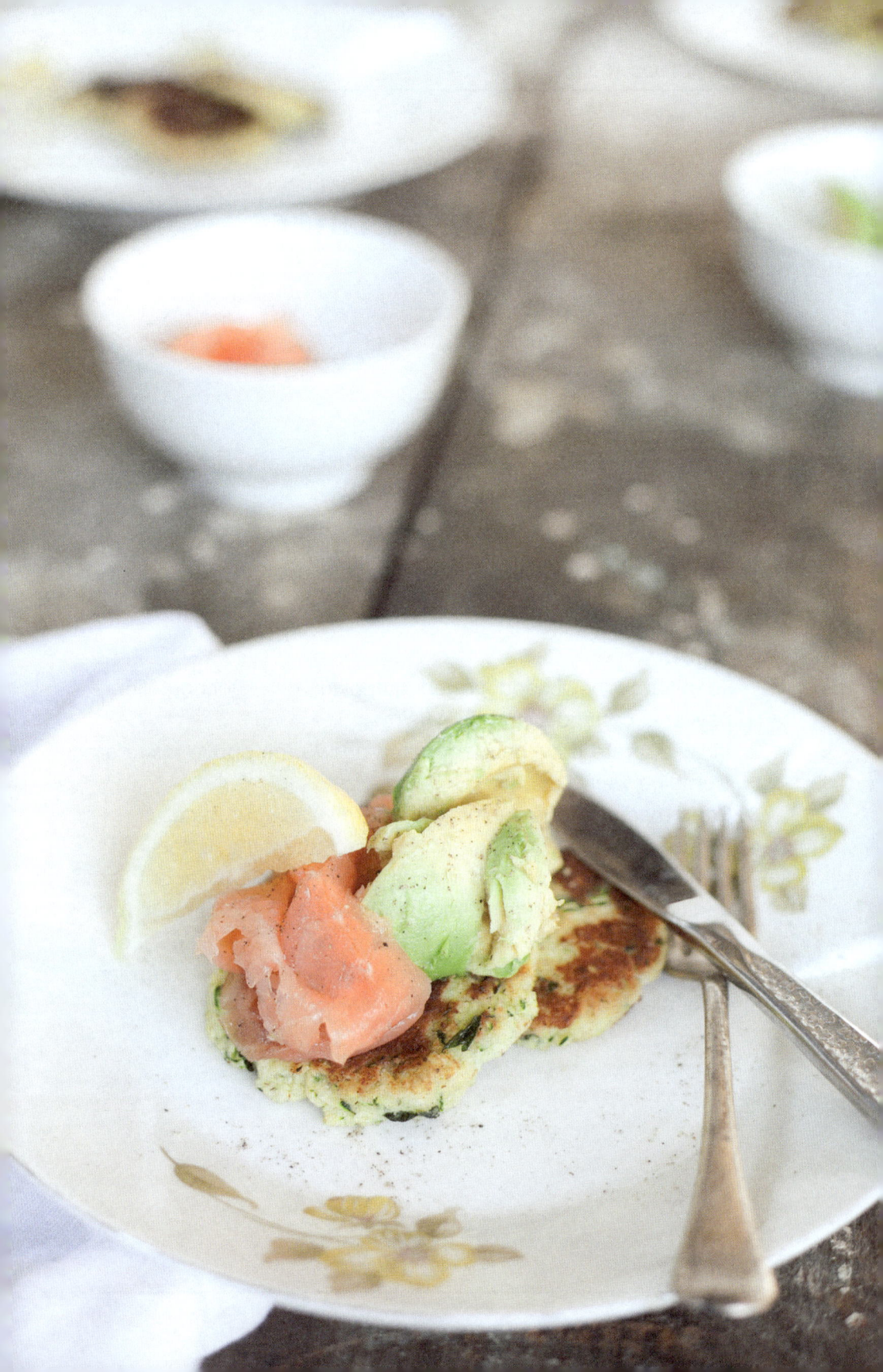

Pumpkin and Feta Fritters

Ingredients (Makes 6)
- 2 cups grated raw pumpkin
- 1/4 cup goat's feta, crumbled
- 1/4 cup coconut flour, sifted
- 1 tablespoon psyllium
- 1 large handful coriander, chopped
- 1 tablespoon chilli flakes
- 2 eggs, free range
- Sea salt and pepper, to taste
- Cold-pressed extra virgin coconut oil, for shallow frying

Method
1. To a large bowl, add grated pumpkin, feta, coconut flour, psyllium, coriander and chilli flakes.
2. In a separate bow, beat eggs and add to the above mixture. Combine well.
3. Form medium balls, molding each well with your hands.
4. Heat coconut oil in a small frypan, flatten the fritters and shallow fry, flipping half way with an egg-flip. Repeat for additional fritters, adding more coconut oil each time. If you are just serving one, you may like to store remaining fritters in the fridge and fry fresh as required. Leftovers will keep for a couple of days.

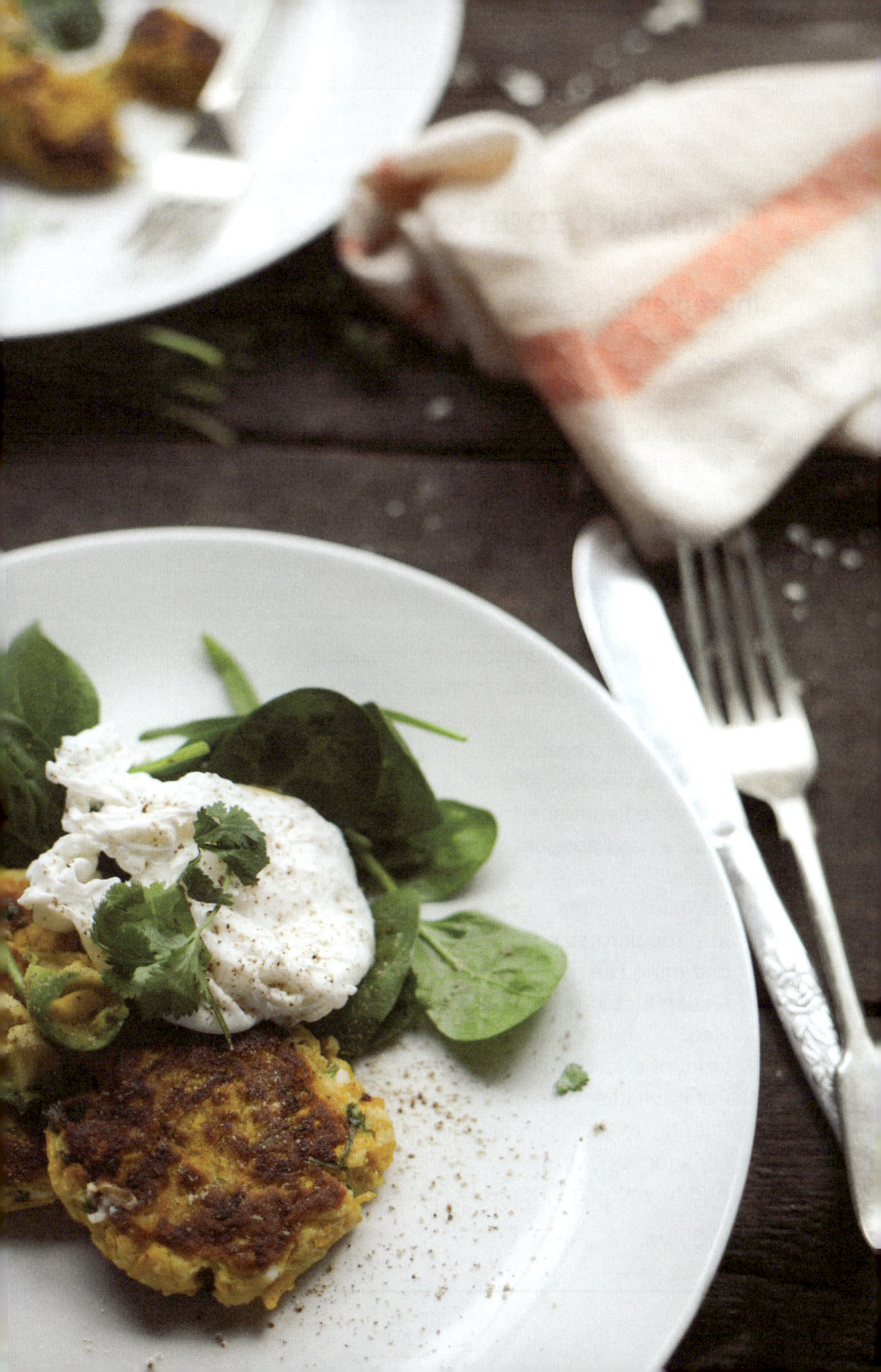

Coconut Crepes

Ingredients (Serves 1)

Crepes:
- 3 eggs, free range
- A dash of unsweetened coconut or almond milk
- 1-2 tablespoons coconut flour, sifted

Fillings:
Option 1
- 1 teaspoon raw cacao
- 1 small handful berries
- 1 sprinkle unsweetened coconut flakes
- 1 teaspoon Pure Harvest organic rice malt syrup

Option 2
- 1/3 zucchini, grated
- 3-4 slices smoked salmon
- 1/2 avocado, mashed
- Sea salt and pepper to taste

Method
1. In a medium sized bowl, whisk together eggs, coconut flour and milk. The mixture should be thick, but pourable.
2. Option 1: add raw cacao; option 2: add grated zucchini.
3. Heat a frying pan over medium heat and melt a small amount of coconut oil in the pan.
4. Pour mixture onto pan, cook until lightly brown and solid enough to flip. Carefully flip with the aid of a spatula and cook for another minute or so.
5. Add to your plate, top with fillings and roll before serving.

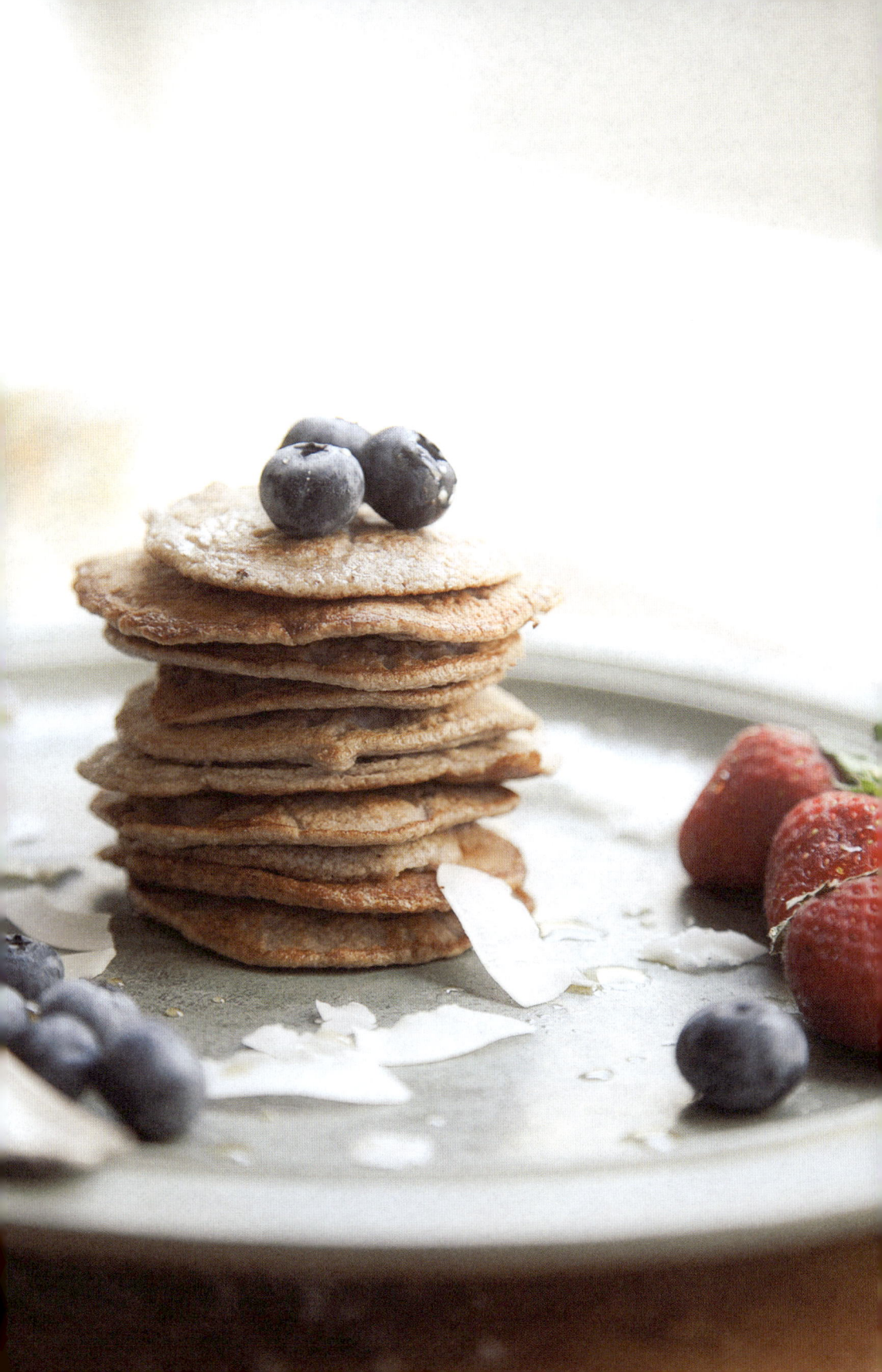

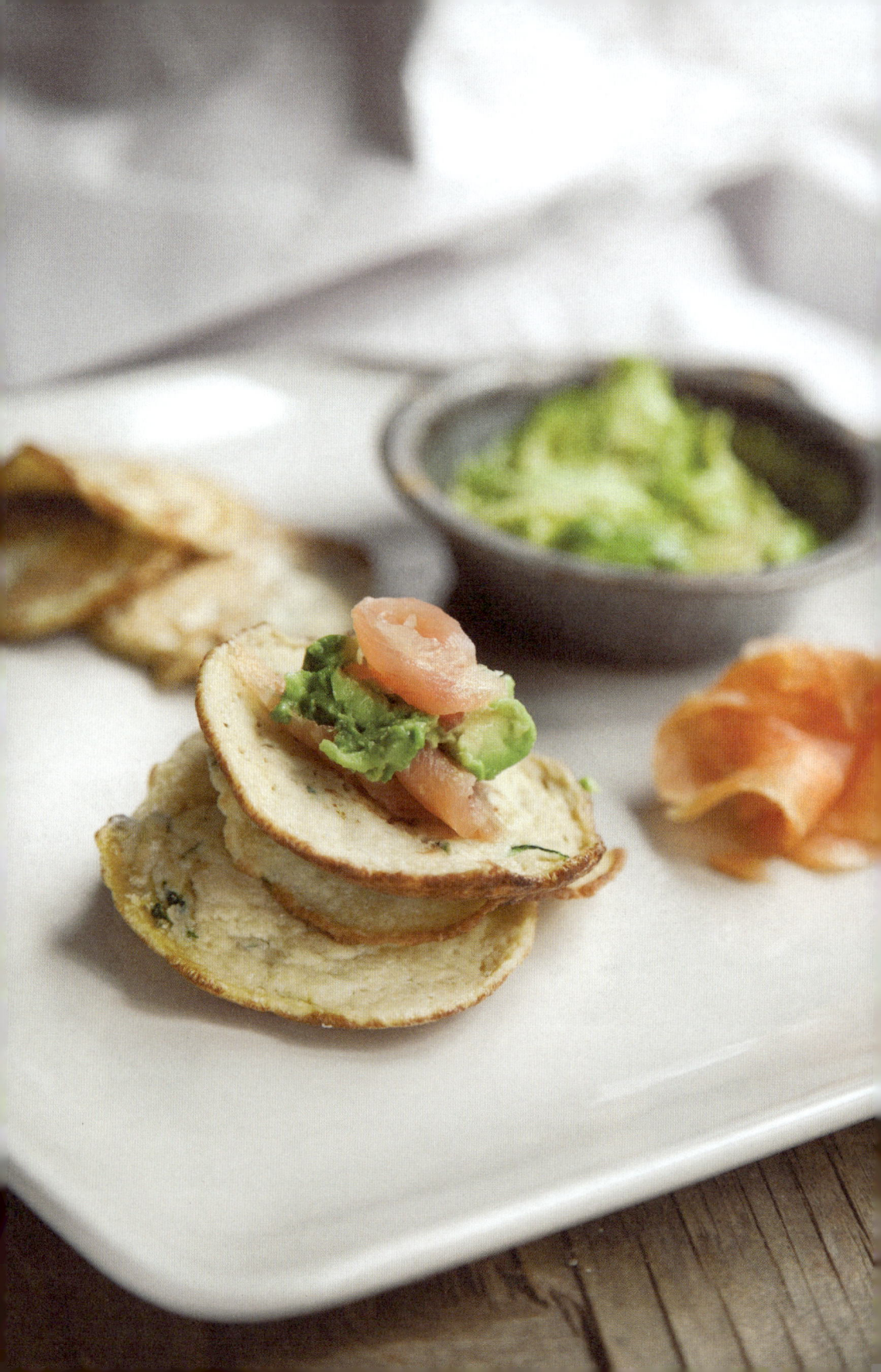

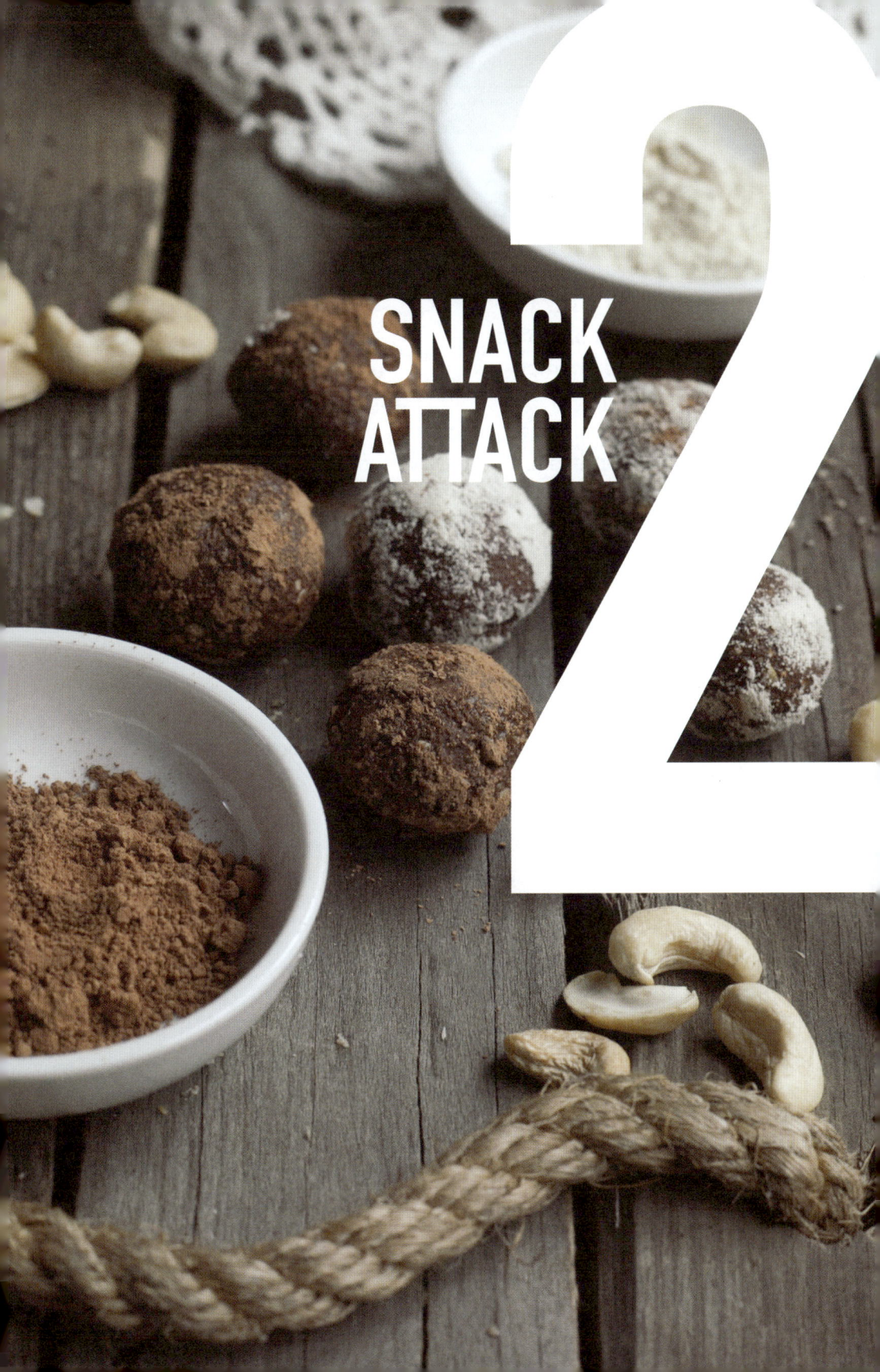

SNACK ATTACK

2

Coconut and Raspberry Delights

Ingredients (Makes 10-12)
- 2 1/2 cups almond meal
- 1 teaspoon cinnamon
- 1 teaspoon gluten free baking powder
- 4 eggs, free range
- 1/4 cup cold-pressed extra virgin coconut oil, melted
- 1/4 cup Natvia
- 1 cup raspberries (fresh or frozen)
- 1/4 cup unsweetened coconut flakes

Method
1. Preheat oven to 160°C.
2. Combine almond meal, cinnamon and baking powder in a large bowl.
3. Add the eggs, oil and Natvia and mix thoroughly.
4. Carefully fold in the berries. Add the coconut flakes and combine.
5. Spoon mixture into lightly greased muffin tins.
6. Bake for approximately 30 minutes or until a skewer inserted comes out clean. Best served warm.

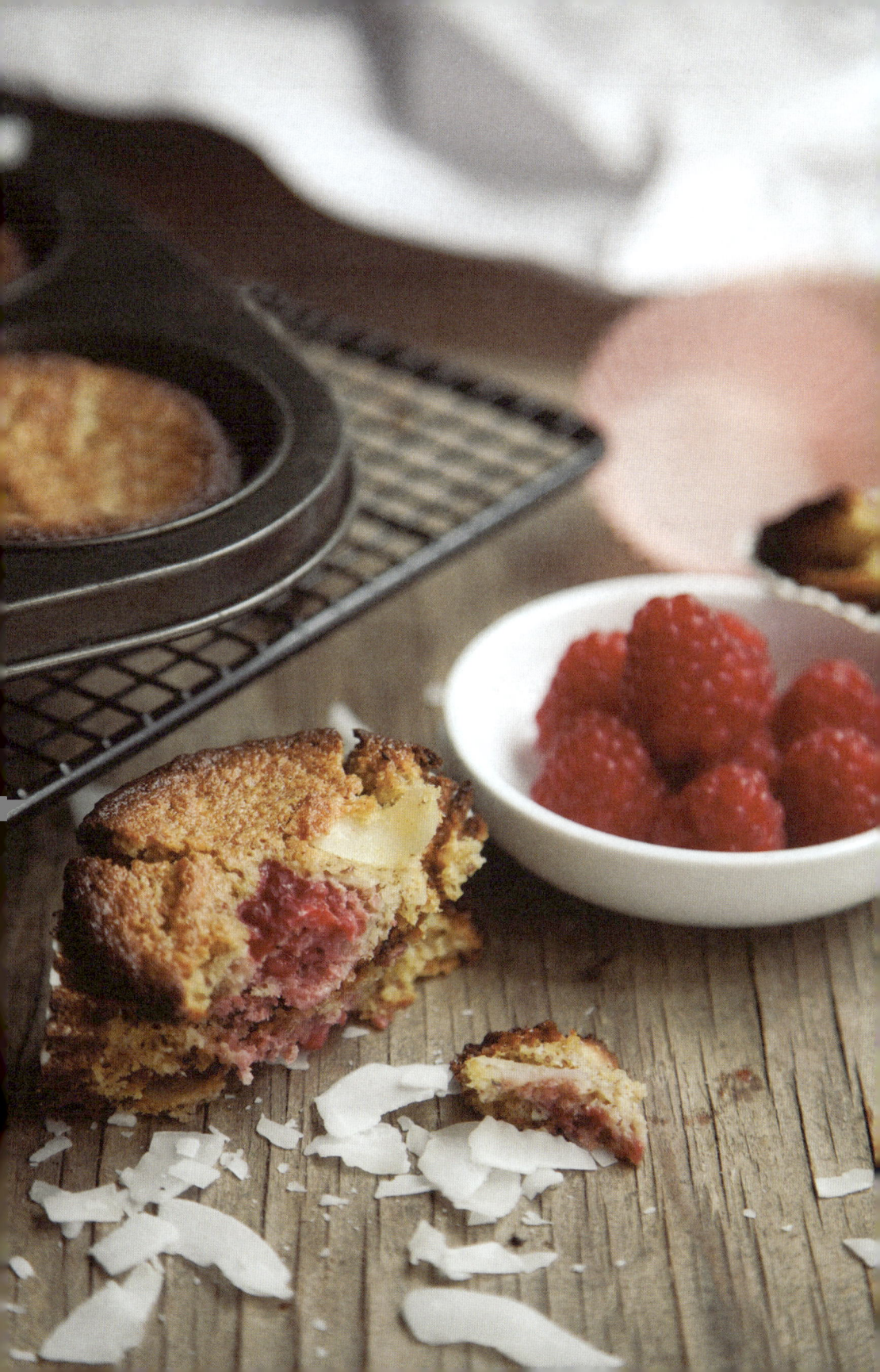

Paleo Zucchini Muffins

Ingredients (Makes 12)
- 2 1/2 cups almond flour
- 1 teaspoon cinnamon
- 2 teaspoons gluten free baking powder
- 1/4 teaspoon sea salt
- 3 eggs, free range
- 1/4 cup cold-pressed extra virgin coconut oil, melted
- 1/4 cup Pure Harvest organic rice malt syrup
- 1 zucchini, grated
- 1 small banana, mashed

Method
1. Preheat oven to 120°C.
2. In a large bowl, combine flour, cinnamon, baking powder and salt. Mix thoroughly.
3. In a separate bowl, beat eggs and add to dry mix.
4. Add oil and rice malt syrup, ensuring all of the dry mix has taken up the liquid.
5. Add the zucchini and banana and combine well.
6. Scoop into a greased muffin tin and bake for 35-40 minutes or until a skewer inserted comes out clean. Best served warm.

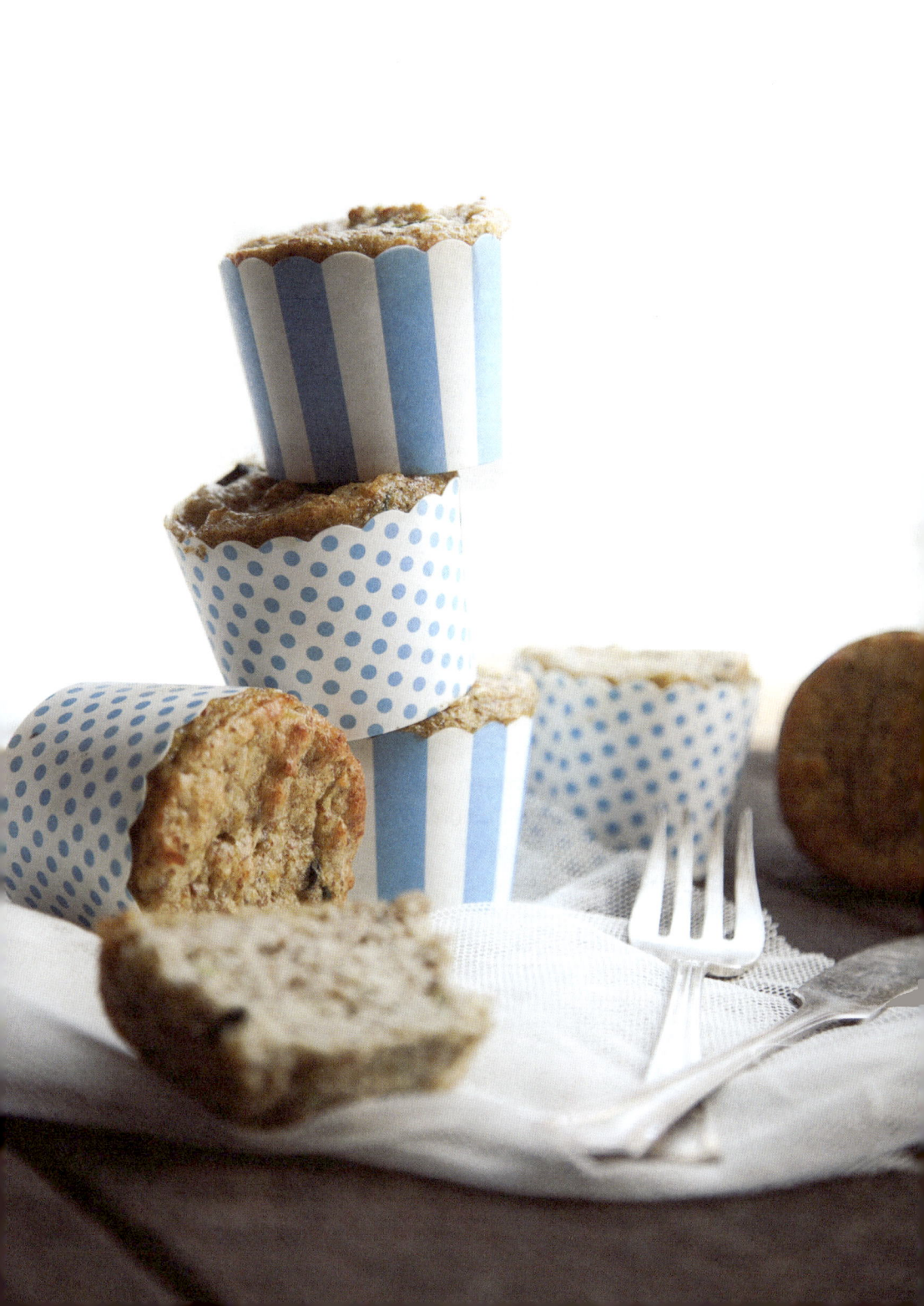

Low Carb Zucchini and Ginger 'Bread'

Ingredients (Makes 10-12 slices)
- 2 cups almond meal
- 1 teaspoon cinnamon
- 1 teaspoon gluten free baking powder
- 1/2 teaspoon sea salt
- 1 tablespoon crystallised ginger, finely diced
- 1 cup zucchini, grated
- 1/4 cup cold-pressed extra virgin coconut oil, melted
- 1/4 cup Pure Harvest organic rice malt syrup
- 2 eggs, free range

Method
1. Preheat oven to 180°C.
2. Combine almond meal, cinnamon, baking powder and cinnamon in bowl.
3. Add zucchini, oil and rice malt and stir thoroughly.
4. Beat eggs in a separate bowl and add to the above mixture.
5. Pour into a lightly greased bread tin.
6. Bake for 20-25 minutes or until golden on top and a skewer inserted comes out clean.
7. Best served warm with a light spread of grass-fed butter.

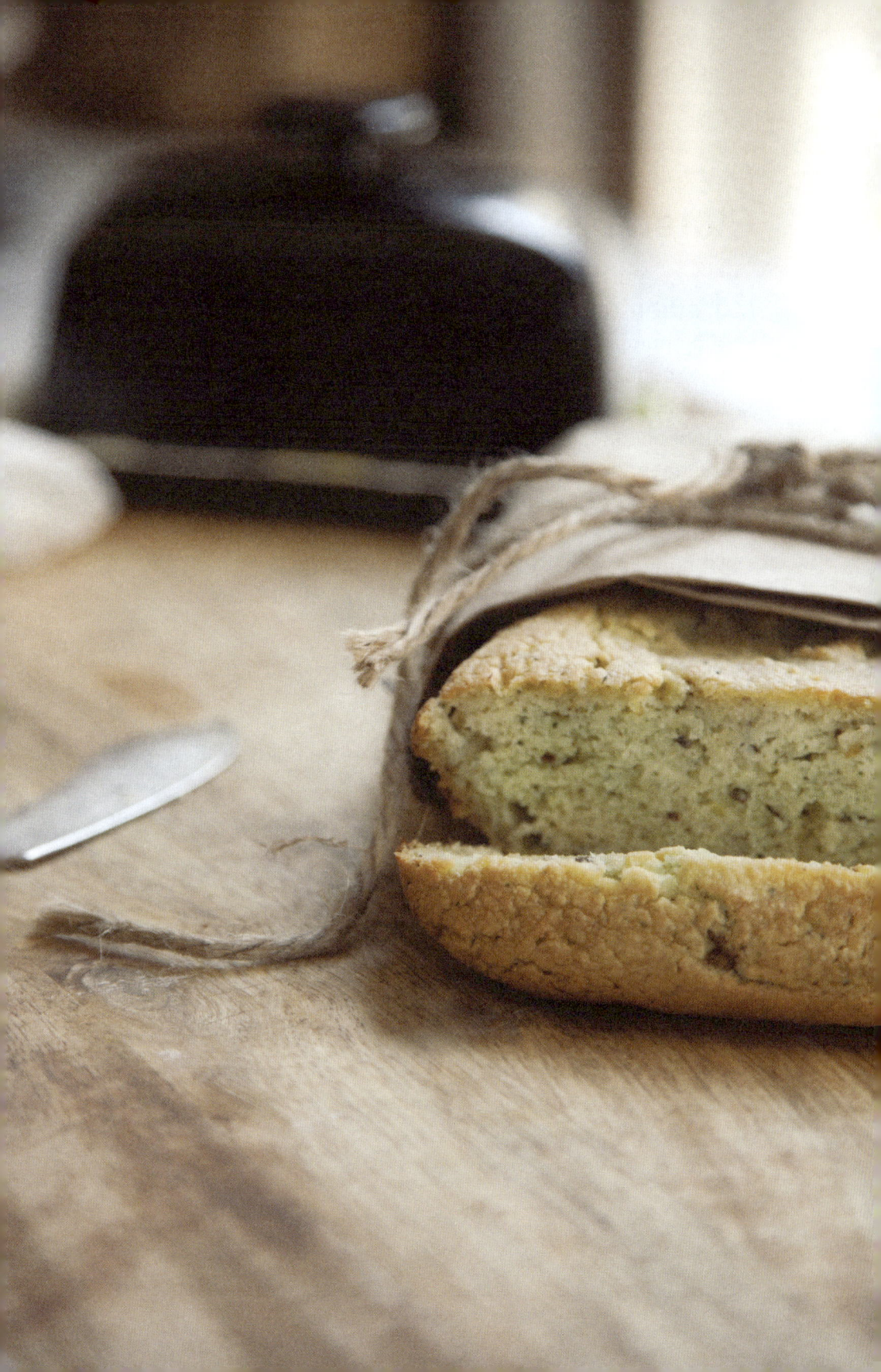

Gluten Free Pumpkin Bread

Ingredients (Makes 10-12 serves)
- 450g pumpkin
- 1 1/2 cups almond meal
- 1 1/2 cups gluten free plain flour
- 2 teaspoons gluten free baking powder
- 1/2 teaspoon sea salt
- 1 tablespoon cinnamon
- 4 eggs, free range
- 1/4 cup cold-pressed extra virgin coconut oil, melted
- 1 tablespoon Pure Harvest organic rice malt syrup
- 1 small handful pumpkin seeds

Method
1. Preheat oven to 180°C.
2. Remove skin and slice pumpkin in small pieces. Steam until soft, mash and set aside to cool.
3. In a large bowl, combine flours, baking powder, salt and cinnamon.
4. In a separate bowl, beat the eggs and add to the flour mix.
5. Add the oil, rice malt syrup and mashed pumpkin and combine thoroughly.
6. Pour into a greased bread tin and spread with extra rice malt syrup before sprinkling with pumpkin seeds.
7. Bake for 1 hour before inserting a skewer to see if it is cooked throughout. If the skewer does not come out clean, leave for another 20-30 minutes before finishing off under the grill. This will obviously be dependent on your oven, so make sure you keep an eye on it after the first hour.

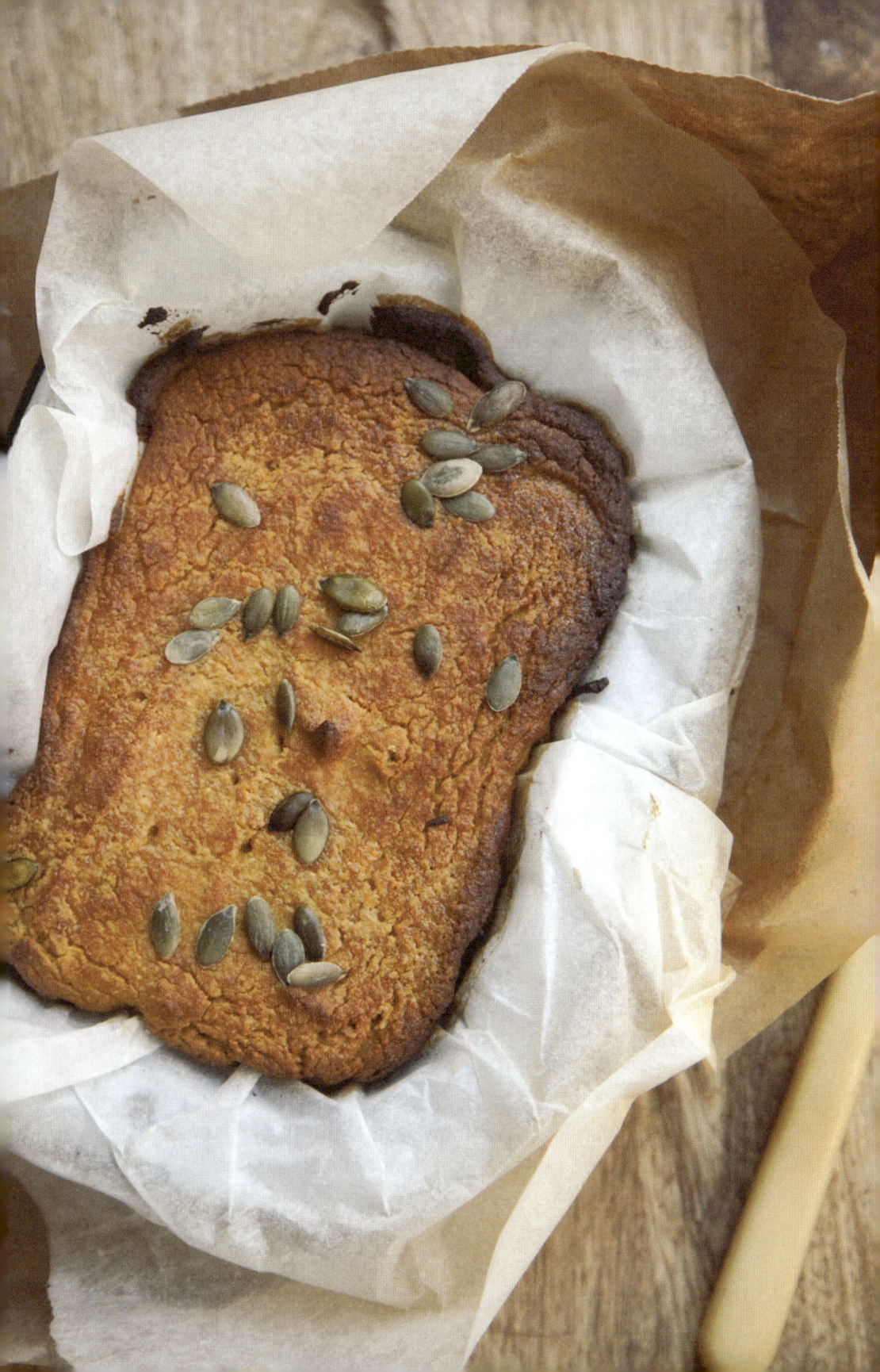

Dairy Free Cashew Pesto

Ingredients
- 3/4 cup raw cashews
- 1 cup fresh basil
- 1/2 cup extra virgin olive oil (EVOO)
- 2 heaped tablespoons nutritional yeast
- The juice of 1/2 lemon, or more to taste

Method
1. Soak 1/2 cup cashews in boiling water for 10-15 minutes or until soft. Drain.
2. Add soaked cashews, basil, EVOO, nutritional yeast and lemon juice and blend until well combined.
3. Add remaining cashews and blitz quickly, depending on desired chunkiness.
4. Taste test and add more lemon juice if required.
5. Serve with chopped carrot and celery.
6. Store in an airtight glass container in the fridge for 5-7 days.

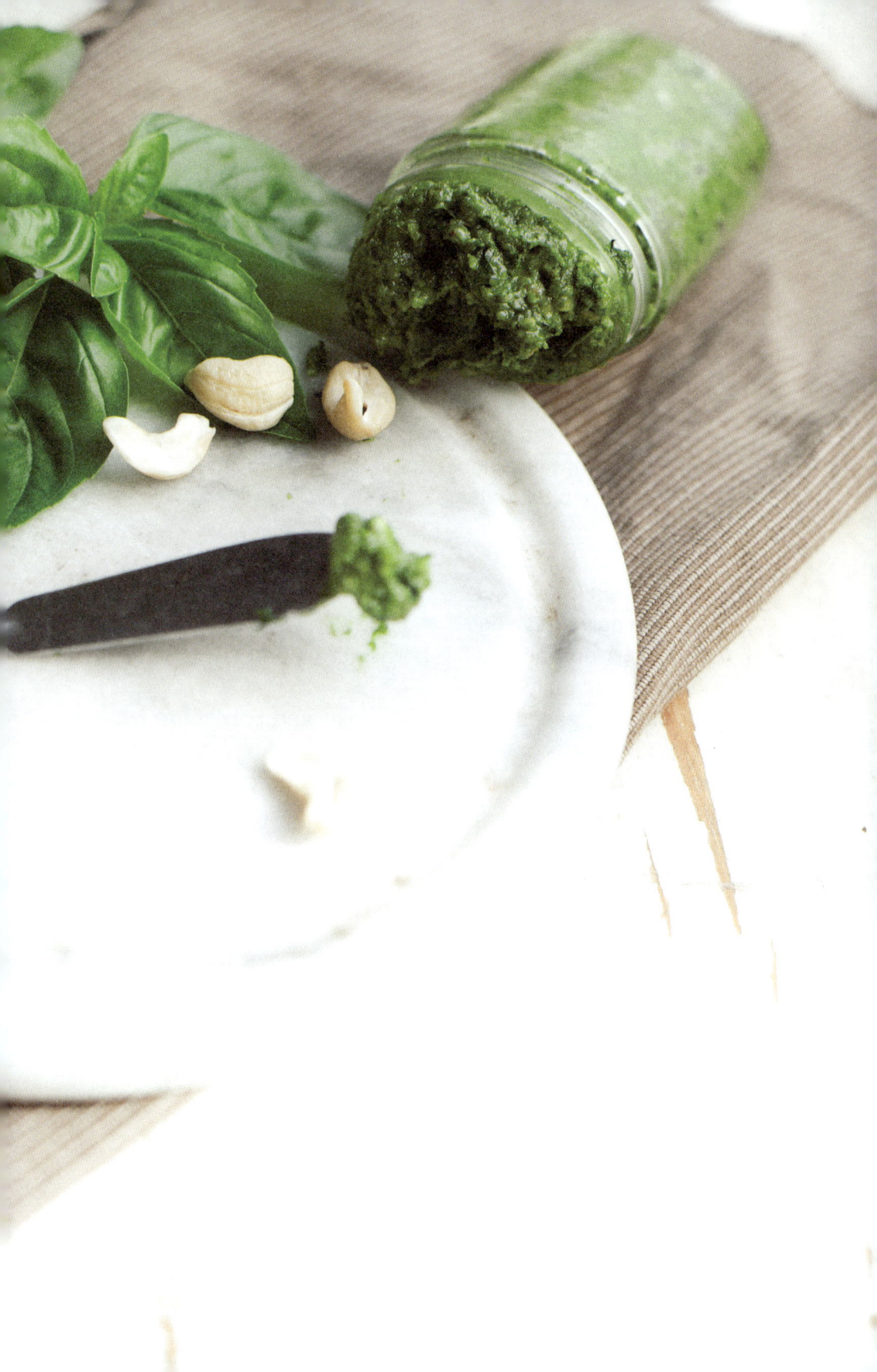

Green Vegie Slice

Ingredients (Serves 4-6)
- 1 zucchini
- 1/2 bunch broccolini
- 5 eggs, free range
- 1/4 cup cold-pressed extra virgin coconut oil
- 1 cup almond or macadamia nut flour
- Sea salt and pepper, to taste

Method
1. Preheat oven to 180°C.
2. Blend or finely chop vegies and add to a large bowl.
3. Whisk eggs and add to the bowl with oil and flour. Stir well and season to taste.
4. Pour into a greased quiche tin or pan and pop in the oven for 20-30 minutes or until cooked throughout.
5. Allow to cool before slicing. Delicious warm or cold and will keep in the fridge for 4-5 days.

Great for a main with sides, as a snack, or even a pre-prepared breakfast idea perhaps?

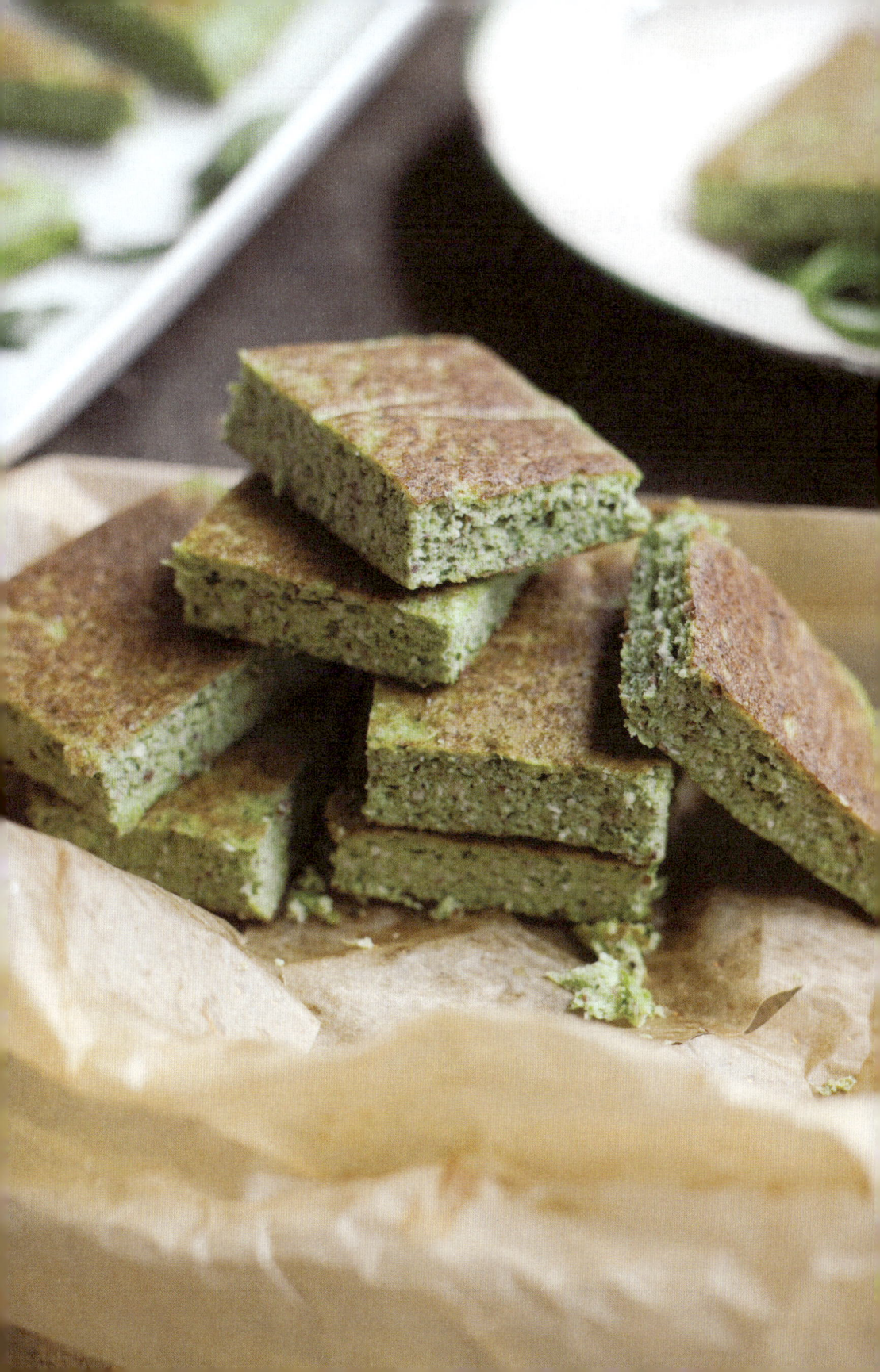

Build Your Own Egg Cups

Ingredients (Makes 10-12)
- 12 eggs, free range
- Sea salt and pepper to taste
- Vegies of your choice
- Goat's feta (optional)
- Cold-pressed extra virgin coconut oil

Method
1. Preheat oven to 180°C.
2. Whisk eggs in a large bowl and season to taste.
3. Pour into lightly greased muffins tins until 3/4 full.
4. Finely chop vegies and add a handful to each muffin tin. If using feta, add a small cube to each cup.
5. Bake for 10 minutes or until cooked throughout. Your egg cups should increase in size and then settle once removed from the oven and allowed to cool.

Packed full of protein, these are fantastic snacks for when you're on the go. You are limited only by your imagination with these.

Some great combinations are:
- Asparagus, spinach and ricotta.
- Bacon, mushroom and sundried tomatoes.
- Sweet potato, broccolini and chilli.
- Mushroom, sundried tomato, capsicum, chive and feta.

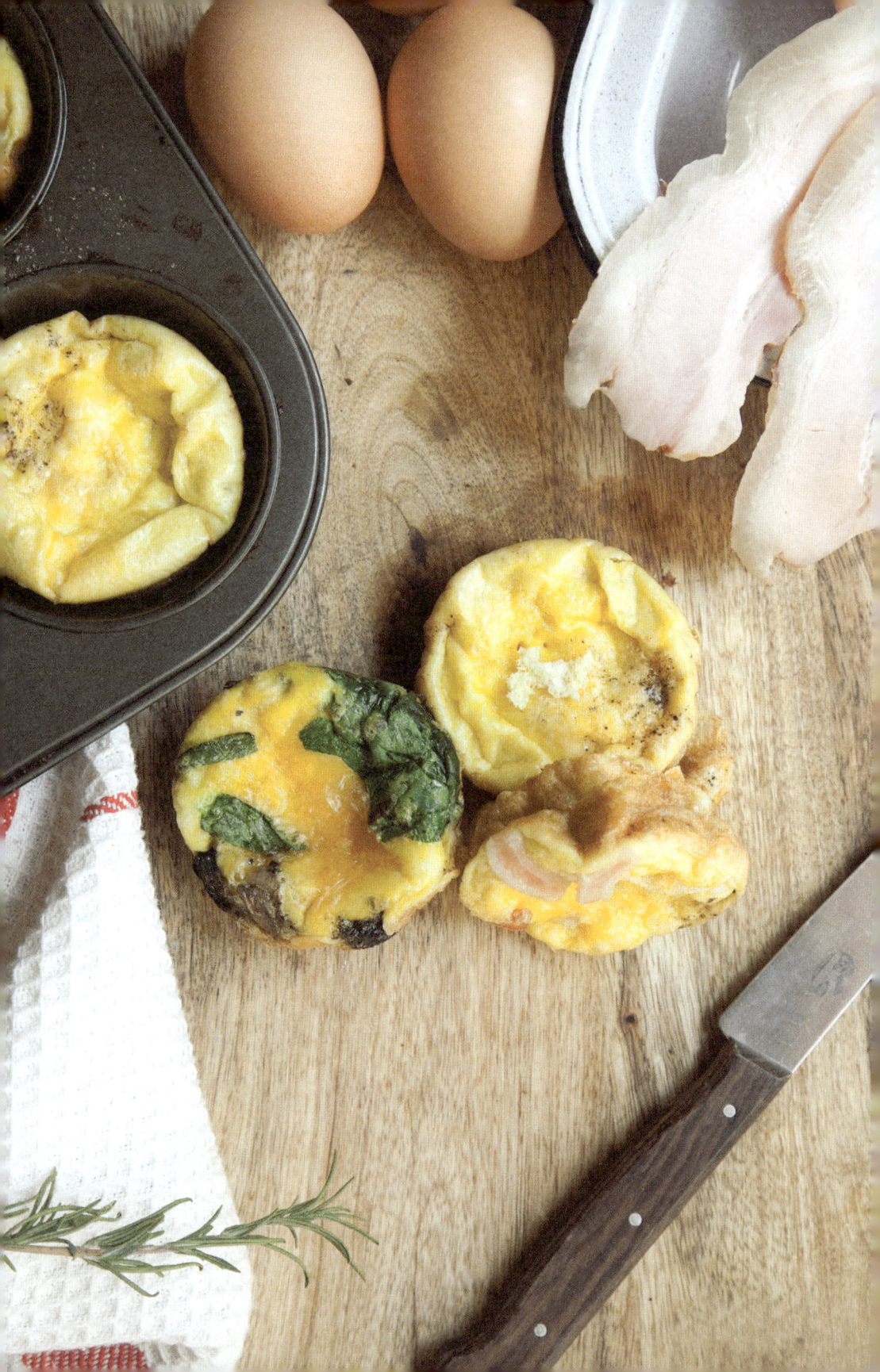

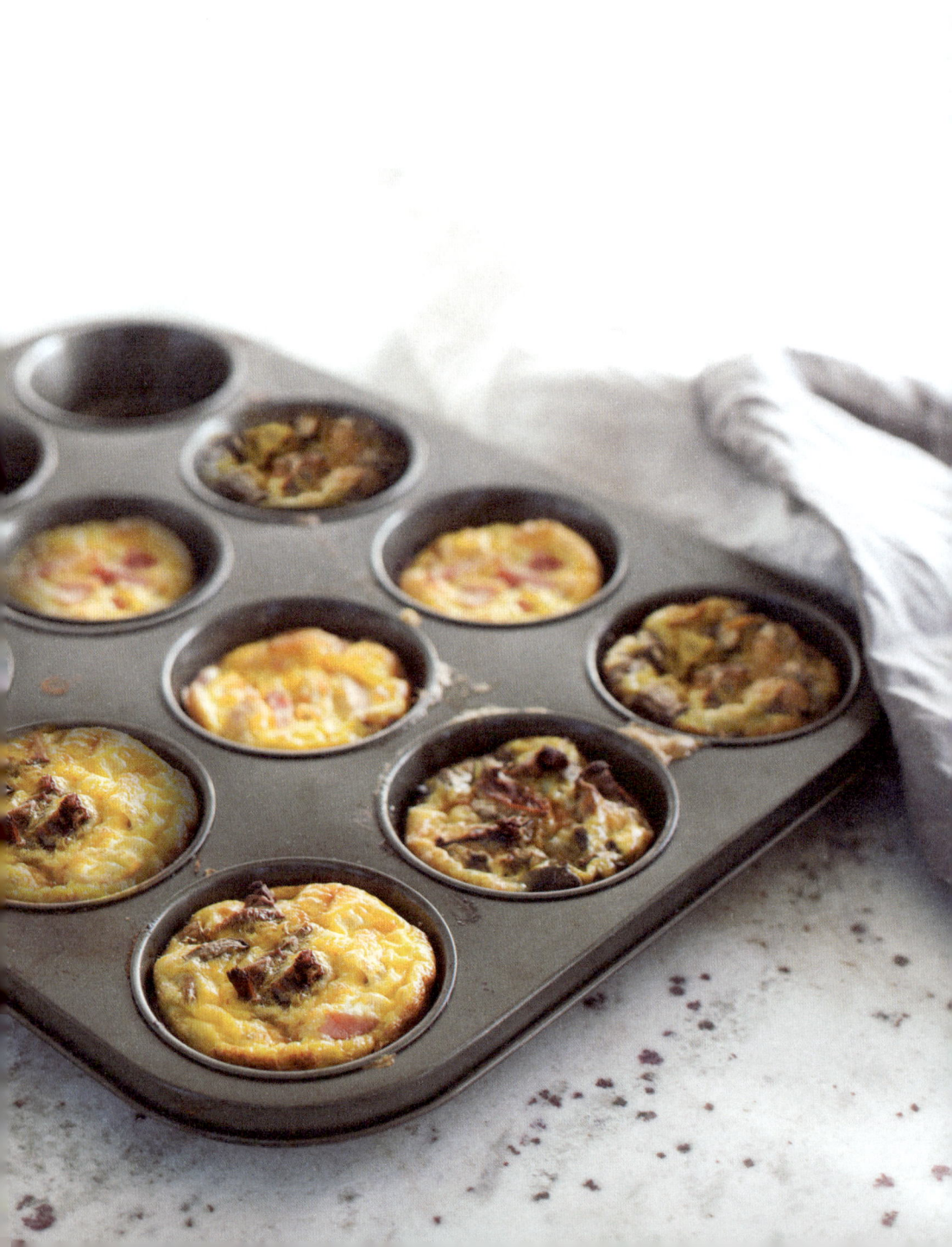

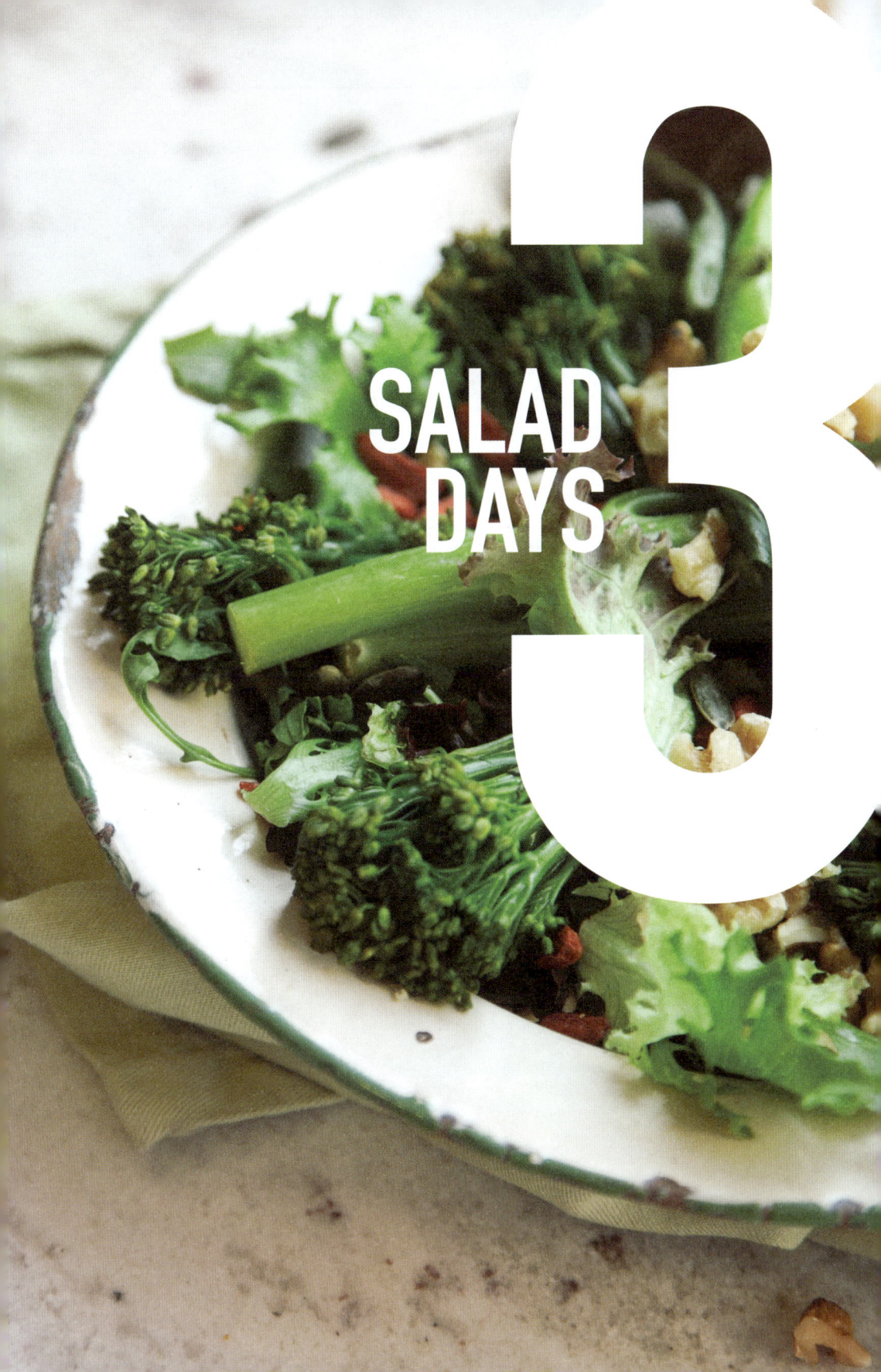

3 SALAD DAYS

Broccoli and Kale Salad

Ingredients (Serves 3-4)
- 2 bunches of broccoli
- 100g kale
- 1 tablespoon cold-pressed extra virgin coconut oil
- 1/2 cup flaked almonds
- 1/4 cup goji berries
- 1/2 large avocado, diced
- 1/4 cup extra virgin olive oil (EVOO)
- The juice of 1/2 lemon
- 1/4 teaspoon sea salt
- Goat's feta to top, optional

Method
1. Dice broccoli heads into small florets and cut the stems into bite size pieces. Lightly steam all and allow to cool in a large mixing bowl.
2. Sauté kale in coconut oil until soft and add to the bowl.
3. Top with almonds, goji berries and avocado.
4. Combine EVOO, lemon juice and salt in a small bowl and dress the salad.
5. Sprinkle with goat's feta and serve with your choice of protein. Leftovers are perfect for lunch the next day.

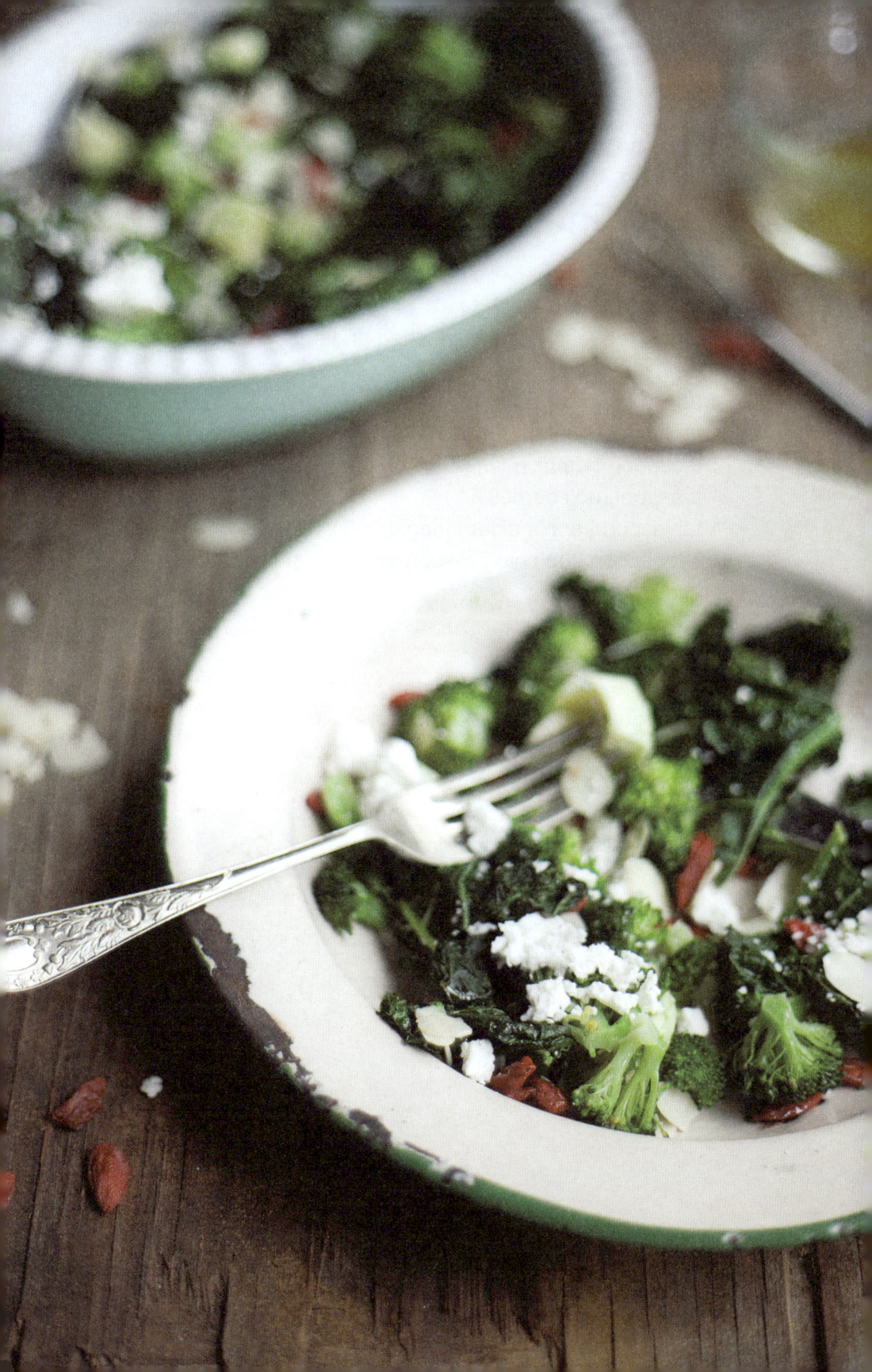

Broccolini Beauty

Ingredients (Serves 1)
- 150g mixed leafy greens, washed and patted dry
- ½ avocado, chopped
- 1 bunch broccolini
- 1 tablespoon walnuts, chopped
- 1 teaspoon pumpkin seeds
- 1 teaspoon goji berries
- 1 tablespoon apple cider vinegar (ACV)
- 1 tablespoon cup cold-pressed extra virgin coconut oil, melted

Method
1. Lightly steam the broccolini and set aside to cool.
2. In a large bowl, arrange the salad leaves.
3. Add the avocado and carefully fold through.
4. Lay the broccolini on top.
5. Sprinkle with the nuts, seeds and berries.
6. Dress with the ACV and coconut oil.

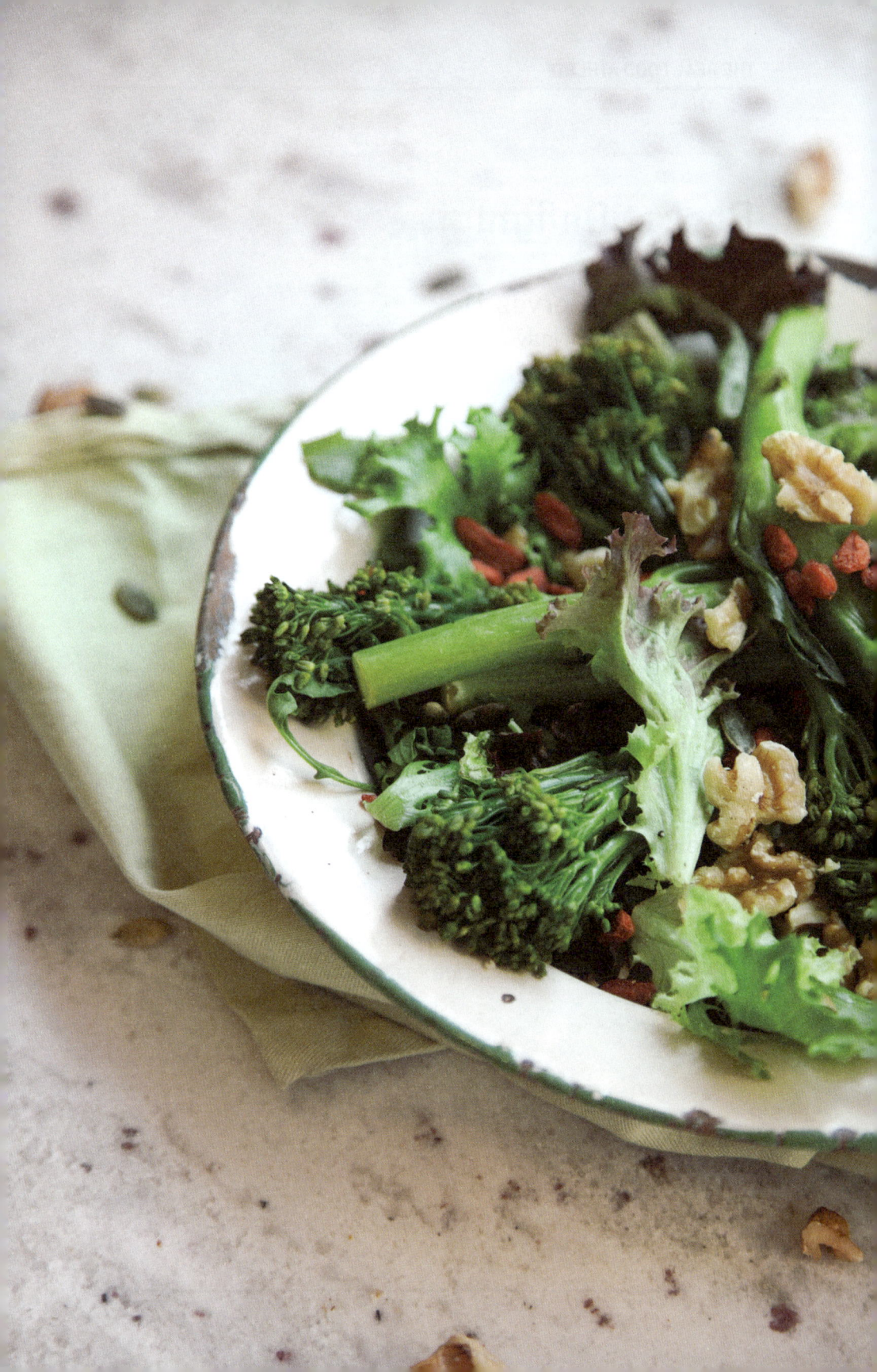

Rocket Delight

Ingredients (Serves 1)
- 1 bunch parsley leaves
- 1 bunch mint leaves
- 1 lemon
- 2 tablespoons extra virgin olive oil (EVOO)
- 2 tablespoon pine nuts
- 150g rocket, washed and patted dry
- 30g goat's feta

Method
1. Finely chop the parsley and mint leaves.
2. Juice the lemon and remove the rind with a grater.
3. To make the dressing, combine the parsley, mint, lemon juice and zest with half the olive oil in a blender, food processor or bar mix. Set aside.
4. Lightly toast the pine nuts and toss through the rocket in a large bowl.
5. Dress the rocket mix with the pre-made dressing.
6. Crumble feta on top.

This dressing is a fantastic addition to any salad. Make extra in advance and store in the fridge for up to a week.

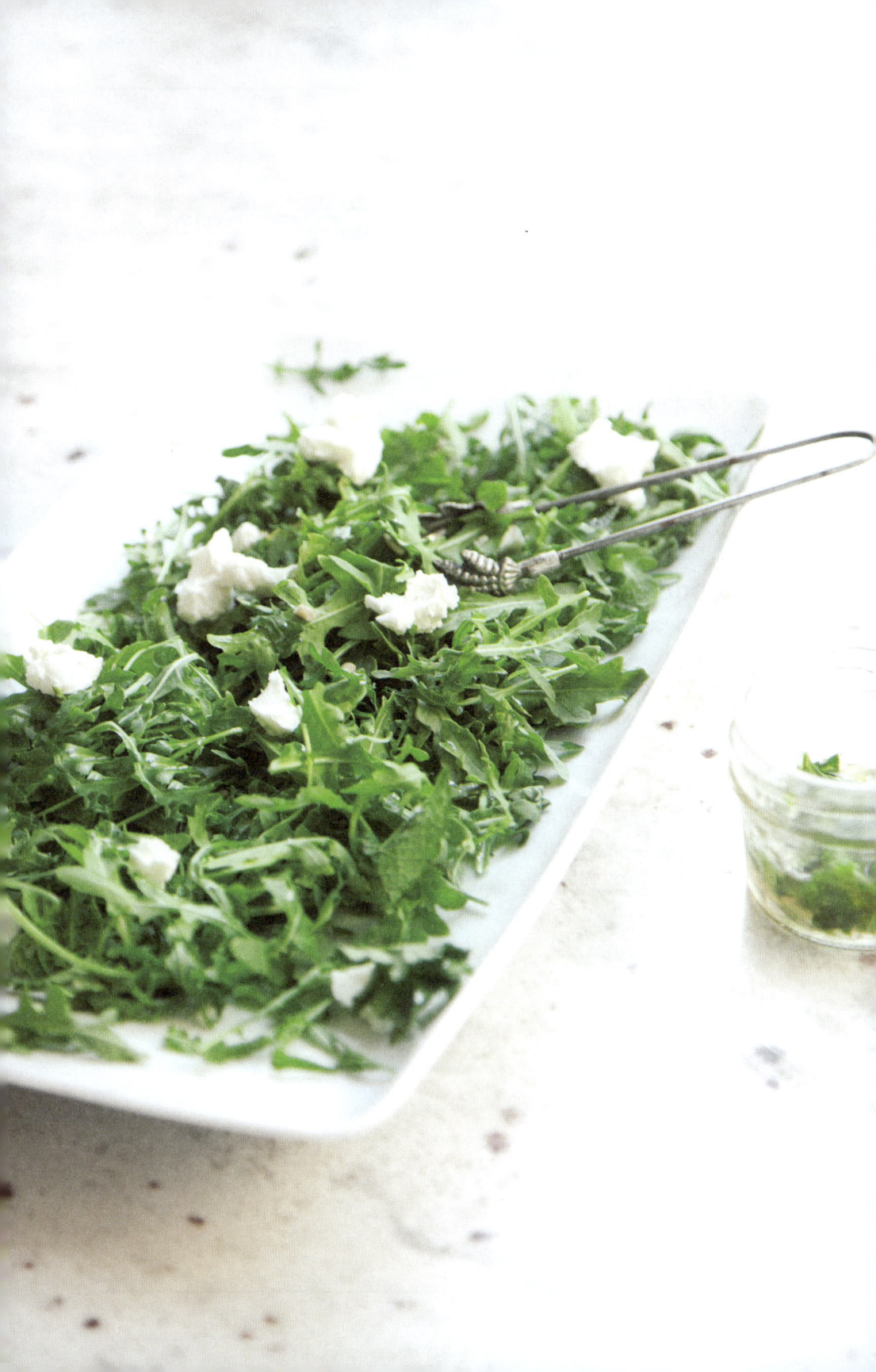

Warm Fennel and Cauliflower Salad

Ingredients (Serves 1)
- 1/2 small cauliflower
- 1 small fennel bulb
- 1 tablespoon extra virgin olive oil (EVOO)
- 1 teaspoon cumin
- 1 teaspoon paprika
- 1/2 teaspoon garlic powder
- 1/2 teaspoon sea salt

Method
1. Preheat oven to 180°C.
2. Wash and cut cauliflower into florets and fennel into quarters.
3. In a large mixing bowl combine remaining ingredients.
4. Toss cauliflower and fennel through until each piece is coated well.
5. Place on a baking try and roast in the oven for 20 minutes.
6. Flip and continue to roast for another 20 minutes or until golden brown.

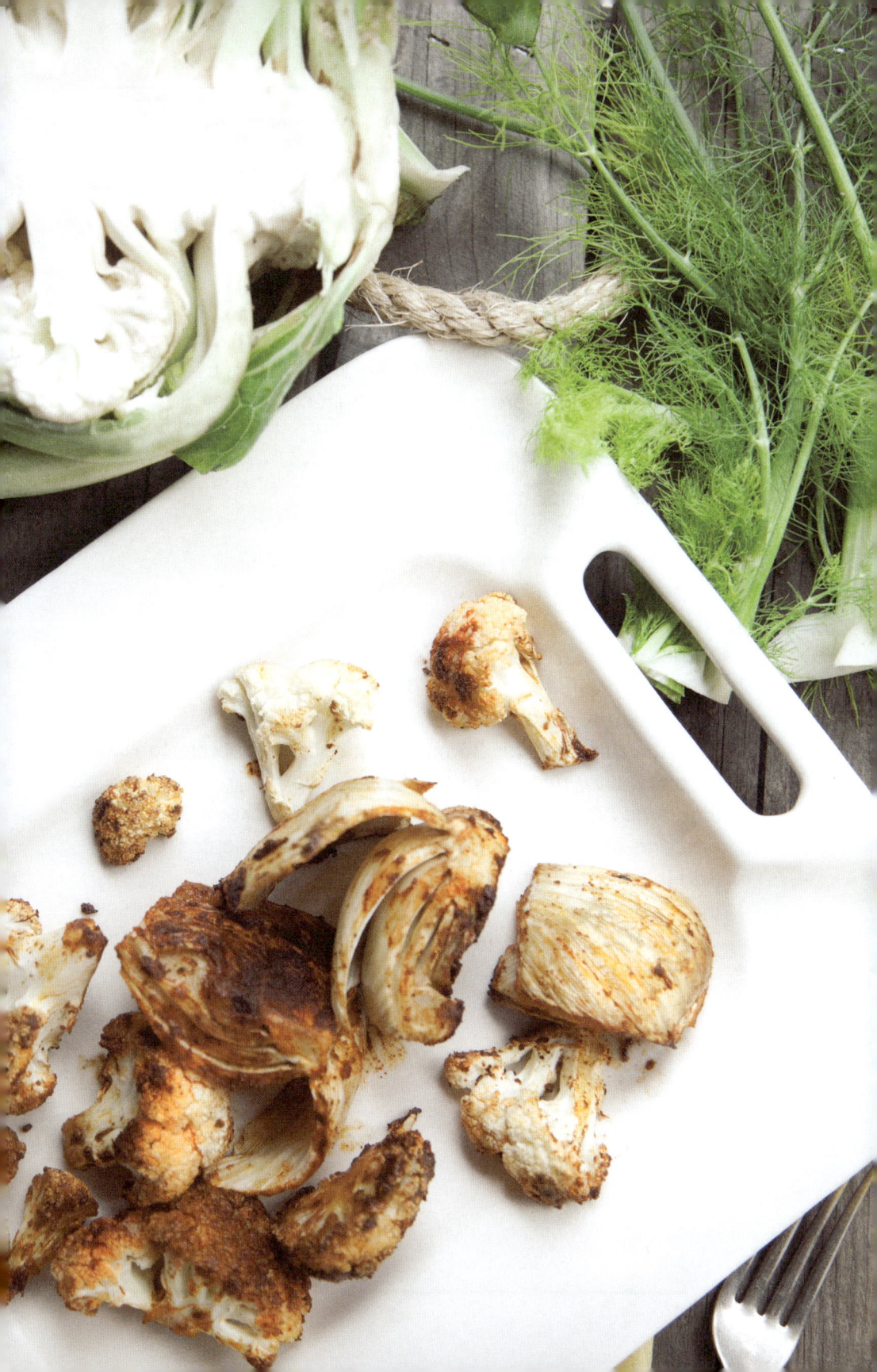

Pumpkin and Purple Cabbage Salad

Ingredients (Serves 1)
- 1/4 small pumpkin
- 2 tablespoons cold-pressed extra virgin coconut oil
- 1/4 purple cabbage, finely chopped
- 1 large handful of spinach and rocket mix
- 1 teaspoon pumpkin seeds
- 1 tablespoon tamari
- 2 tablespoons lemon juice, freshly squeezed

Method
1. Preheat oven to 180°C.
2. Chop pumpkin, place on a baking tray and cover with 1 tablespoon of coconut oil.
3. Roast in the oven for 20 minutes, flip and continue to roast for another 20 minutes or until golden brown.
4. In a large bowl, combine the spinach and rocket mix with the cabbage and pumpkin seeds.
5. Add the roast pumpkin and combine thoroughly.
6. In a separate bowl, combine the tamari and lemon juice. Dress the salad to taste.

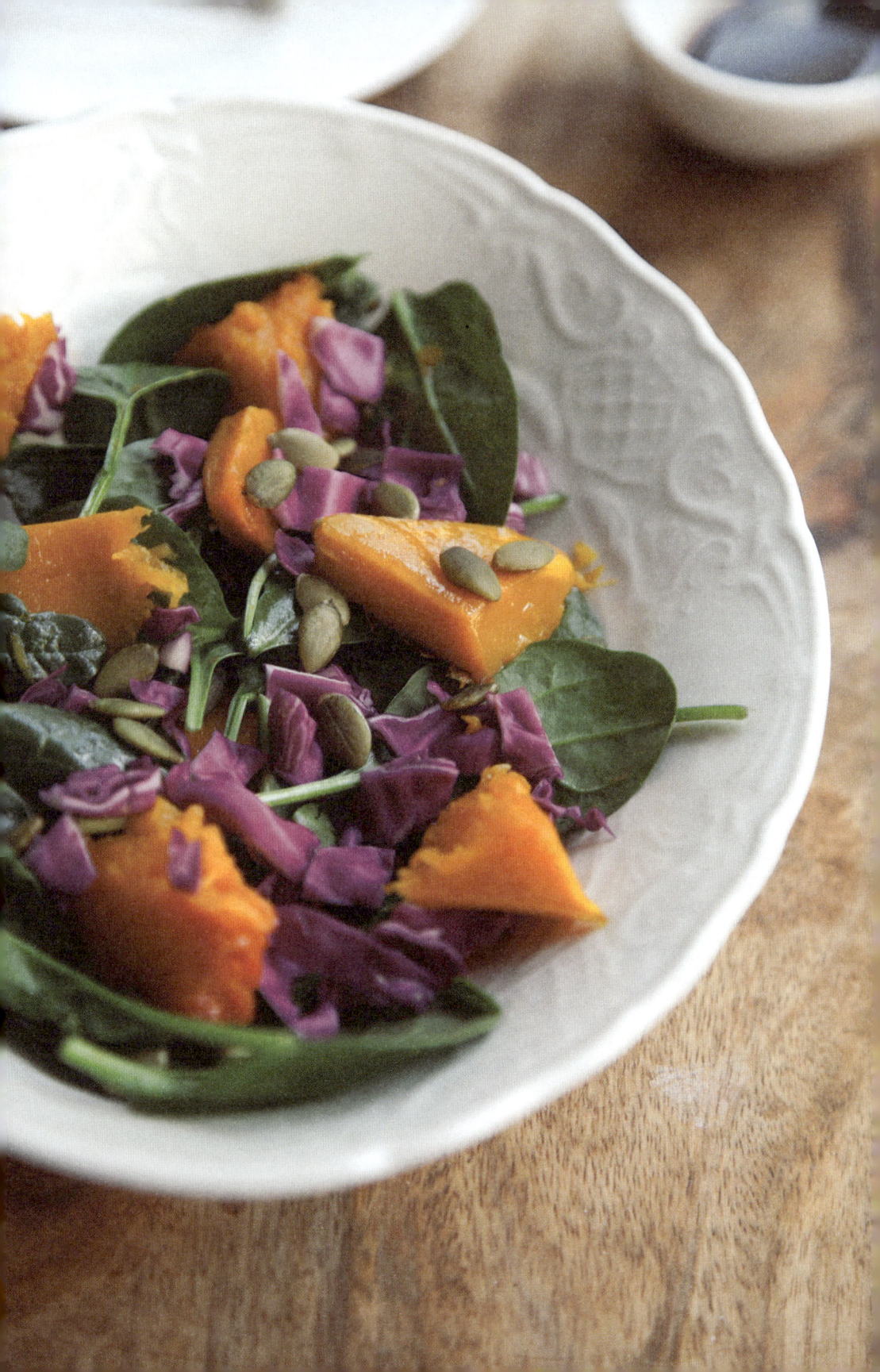

Superfood Salad

Ingredients (Serves 1)
- 1/2 cup quinoa
- 1 handful spinach
- 1/2 cup fennel, finely chopped
- 1 tablespoon apple cider vinegar (ACV)
- 2 tablespoons extra virgin olive oil (EVOO)
- 1/2 pomegranate, seeded
- 1 teaspoon pumpkin seeds

Method
1. Bring 1 cup of water to the boil.
2. Add the quinoa and cook until the water evaporates, fluffing halfway through with a fork. Set aside to cool.
3. In a large bowl, thoroughly combine the spinach and fennel.
4. Mix the ACV and EVOO together in a small bowl and dress the greens.
5. Stir through 2 tablespoons of the cooked quinoa.
6. Top with the pomegranate and pumpkin seeds.

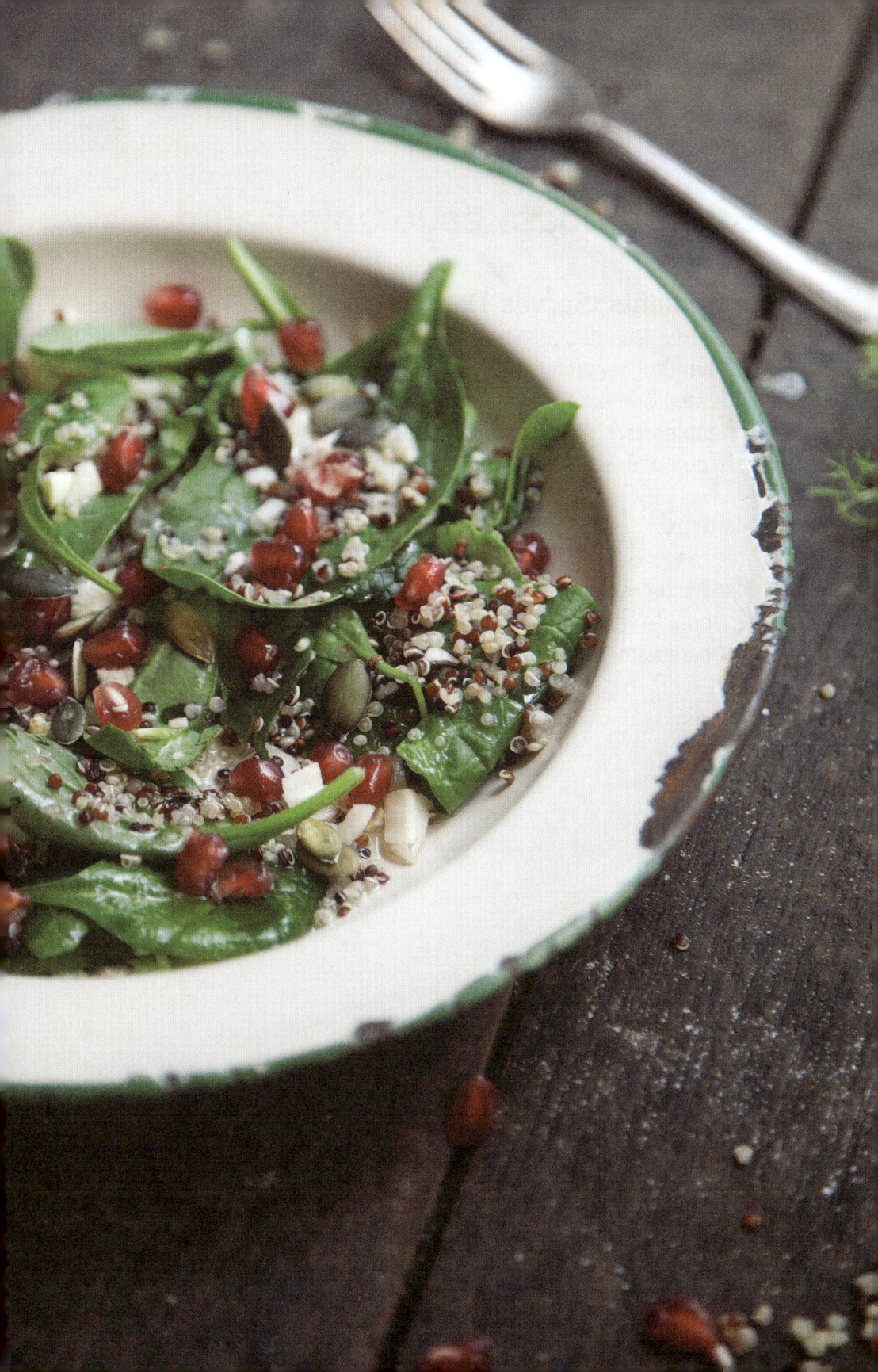

Simple Roast Vegetable Salad

Ingredients (Serves 1)
- 1 serve Roasted Vegies (See 'On the side')
- 1 handful spinach leaves
- 1 teaspoon sunflower seeds
- 1 tablespoon apple cider vinegar (ACV)
- 30g goat's feta (optional)

Method
1. In a large bowl, arrange the spinach leaves.
2. Add the roast vegies.
3. Sprinkle with the sunflower seeds.
4. Dress with ACV and if using, crumble feta on top.

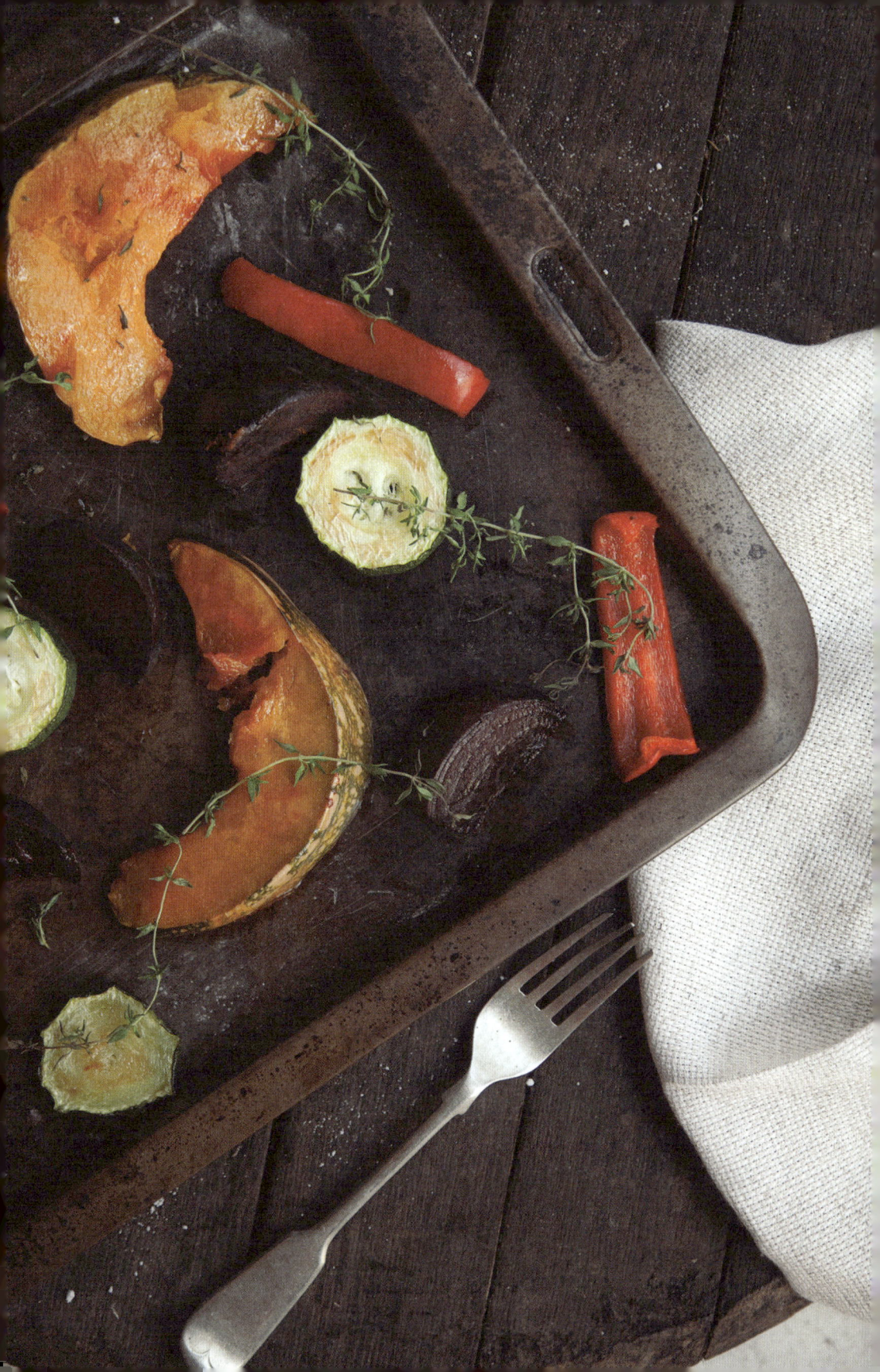

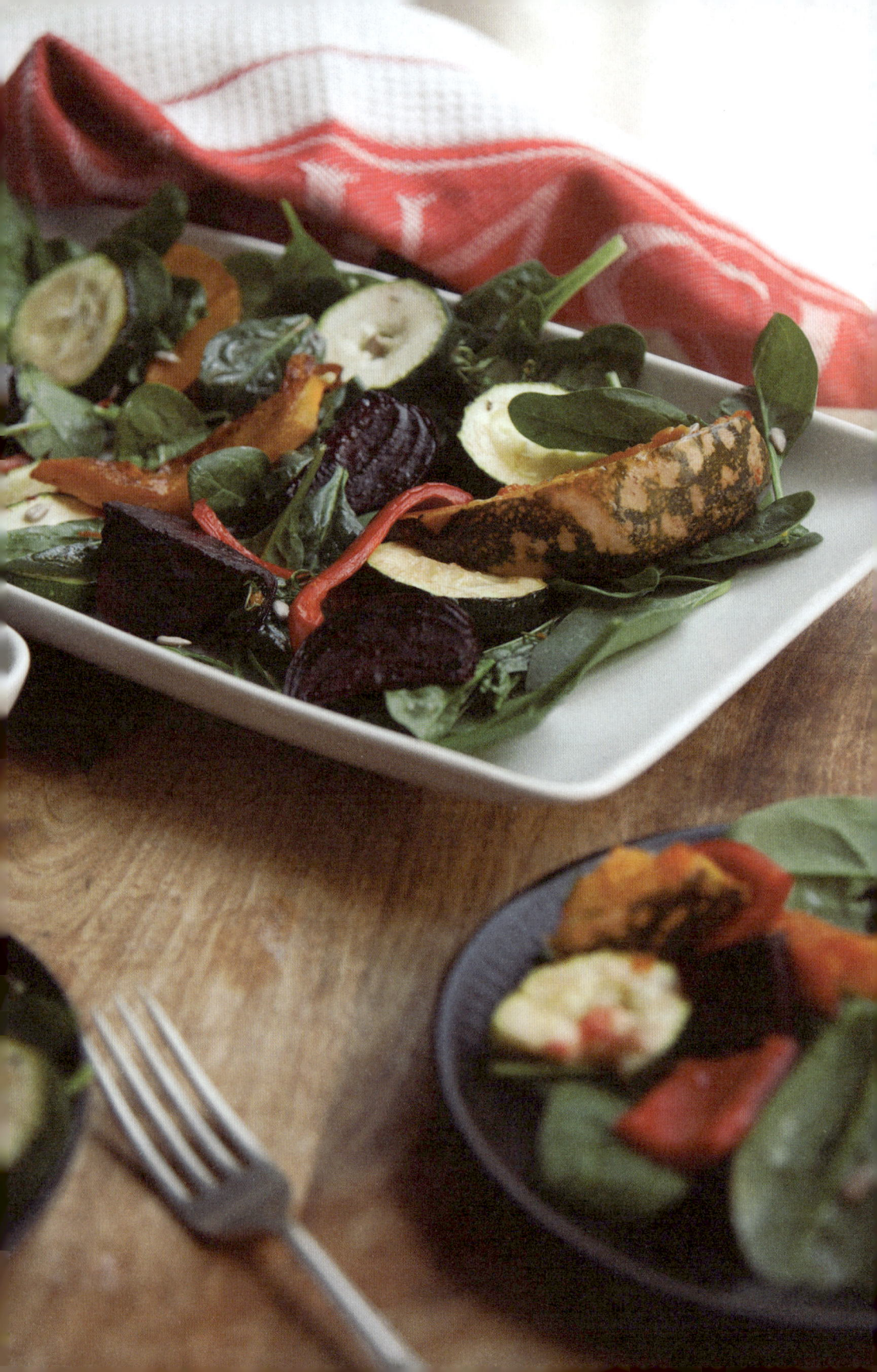

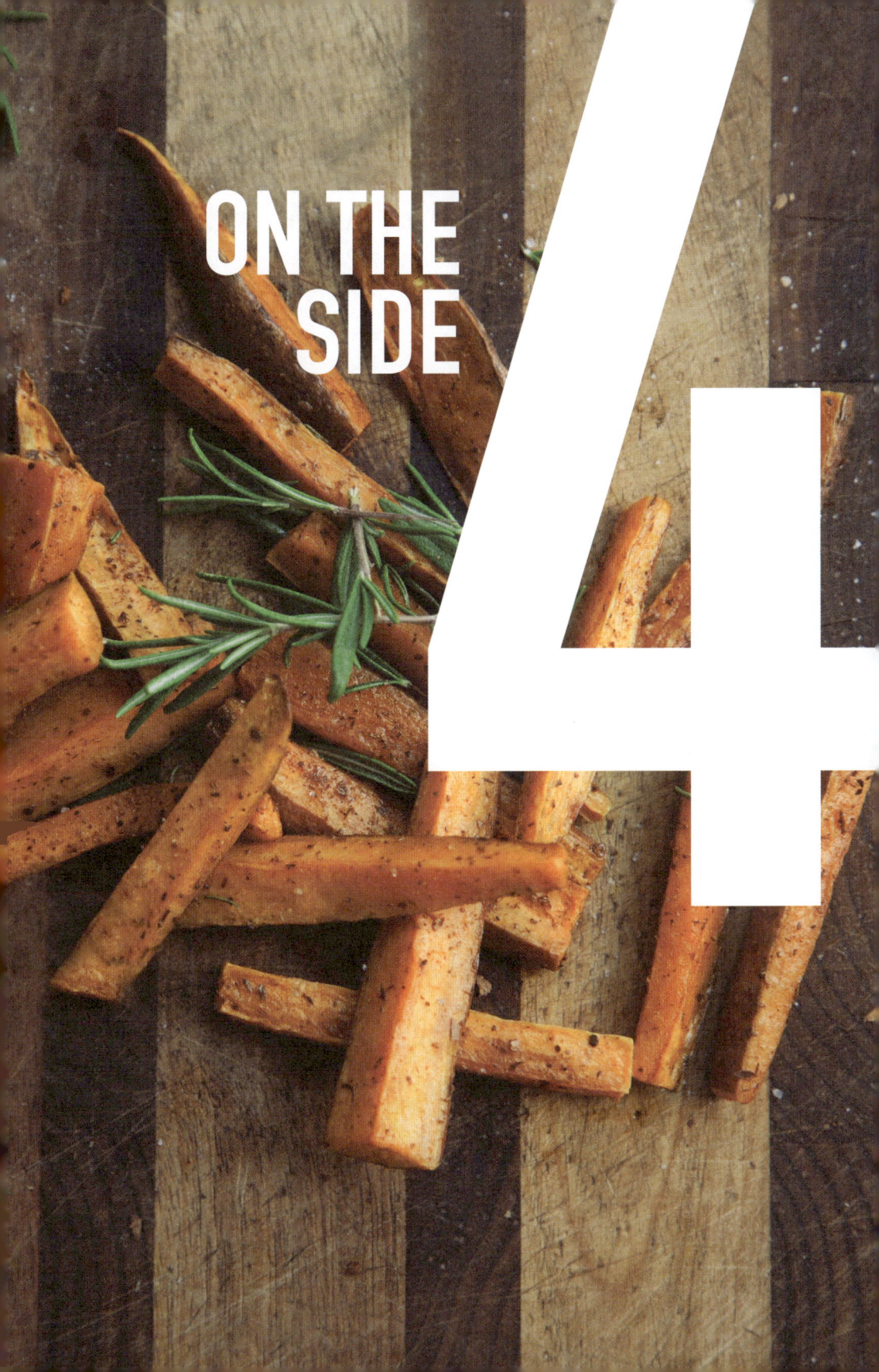

ON THE SIDE

4

Steamed Broccolini with Feta

Ingredients (Serves 1)
- 1/2 bunch broccolini
- 30g goat's feta
- 1 tablespoon apple cider vinegar (ACV)
- 2 tablespoons extra virgin olive oil (EVOO)

Method
1. Lightly steam broccolini.
2. Crumble feta on top and drizzle with ACV and EVOO.

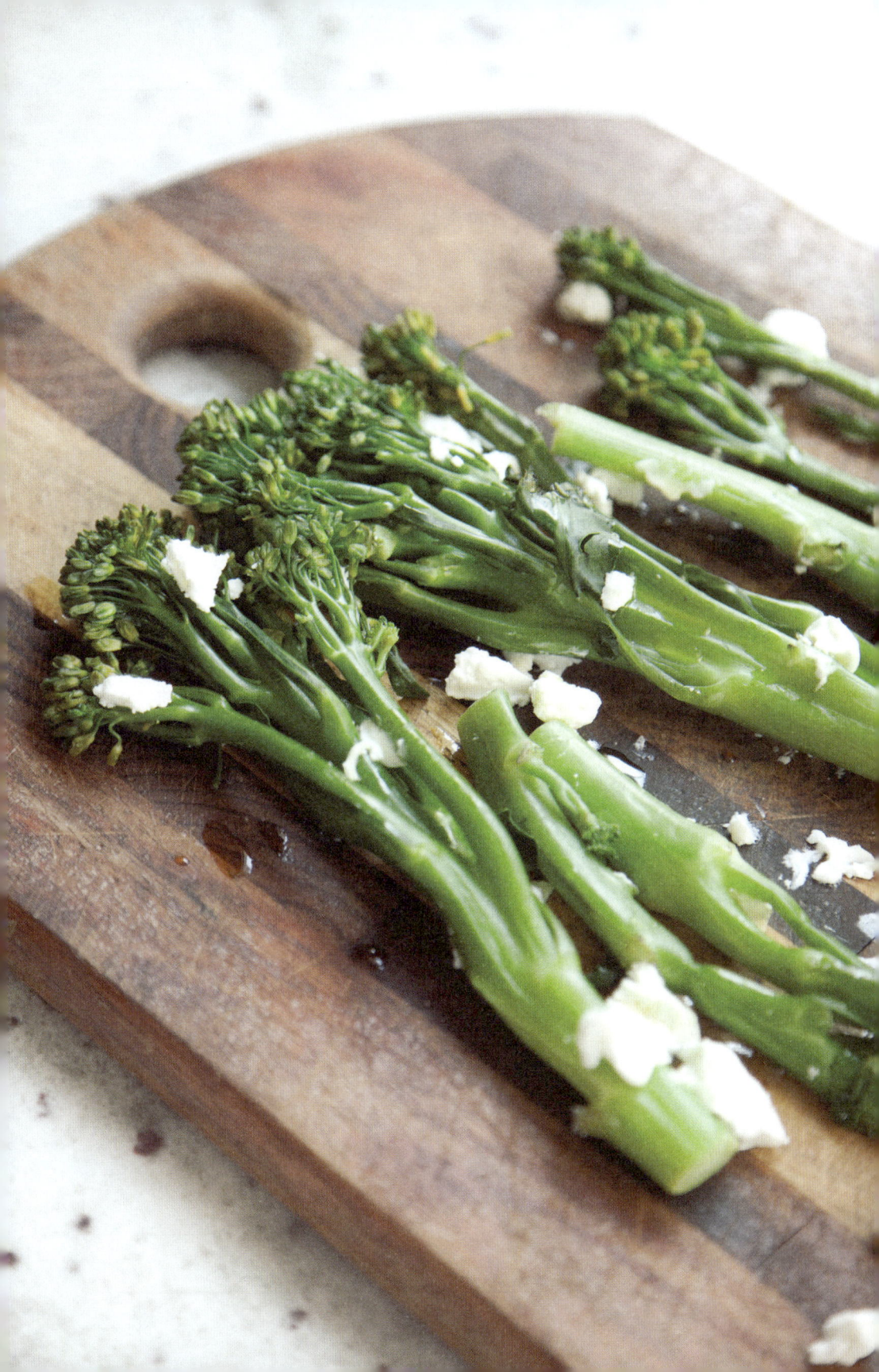

Cauliflower Mash

Ingredients (Serves 2)
- 1 medium cauliflower
- 2 tablespoons grass-fed butter
- Sea salt, to taste

Method
1. Cut cauliflower into small florets and steam until soft.
2. Mash with butter and season with salt to taste.

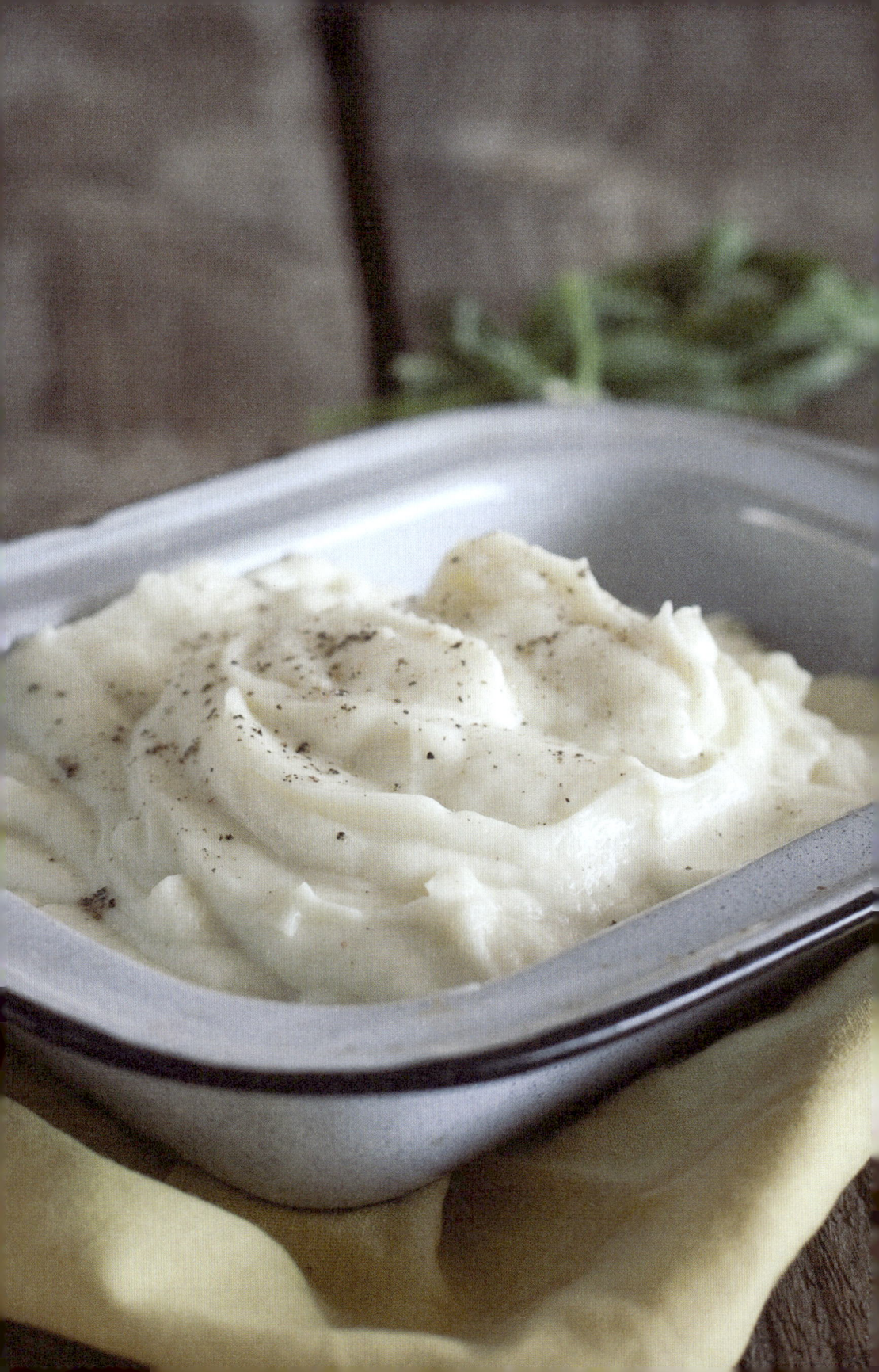

Minted Avocado and Feta Mash

Ingredients (Serves 1)
- ½ avocado
- 30g goat's feta
- 1 small handful fresh mint

Method
1. Mash avocado and feta.
2. Finely crumble fresh mint and stir through.

Perfect with Gluten Free Pumpkin Bread, served with two poached eggs, fresh rocket and lemon.

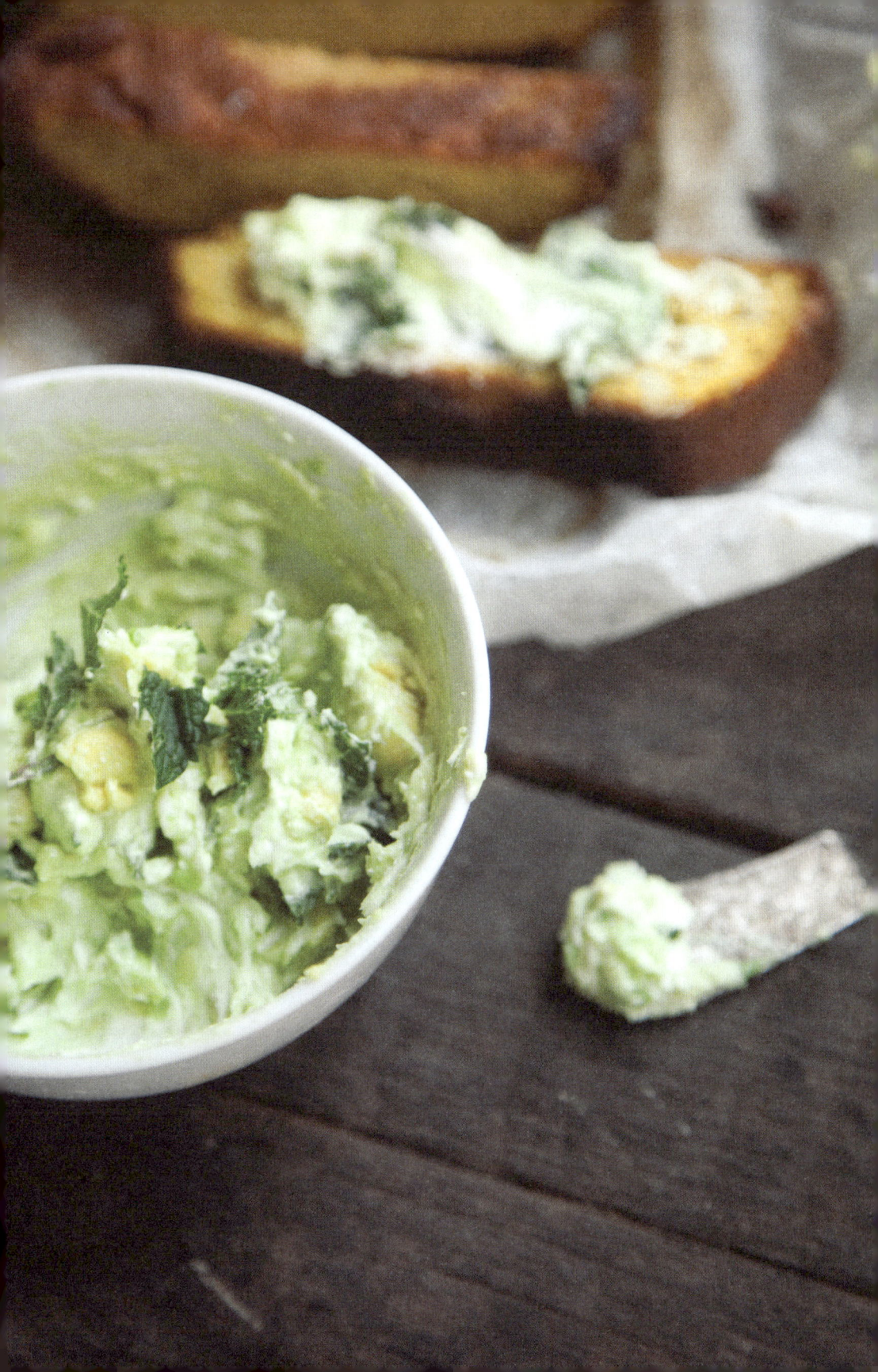

Zucchini Chips

Ingredients (Serves 2)
- 1 large zucchini
- 2 tablespoons cold-pressed extra virgin coconut oil
- Sea salt, to taste

Method
1. Preheat oven to 180°C.
2. Slice zucchini into thin chip-like pieces.
3. Sprinkle with oil and salt and bake for 10-15 minutes.
4. Finish off under the grill until crispy.

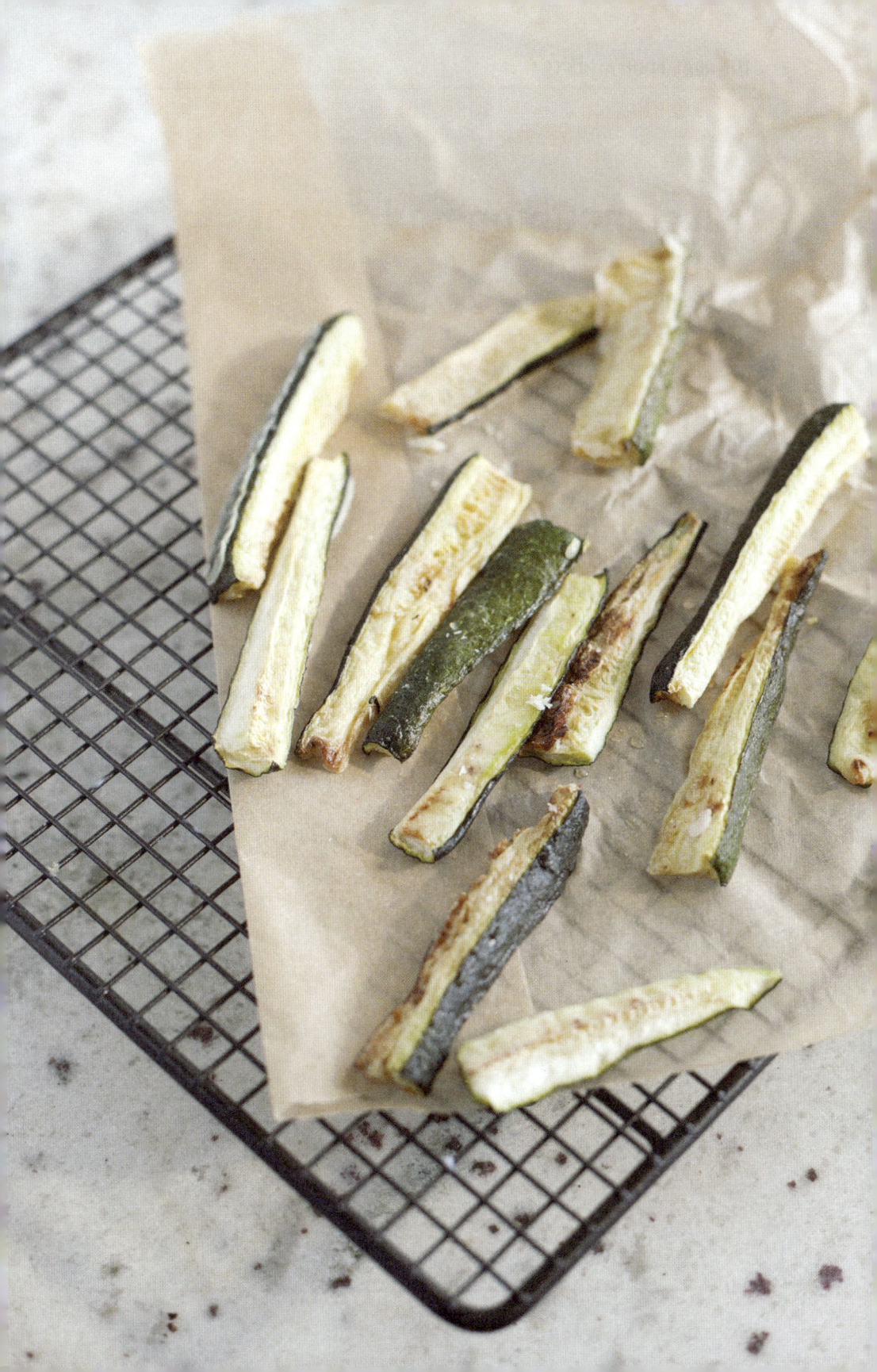

Cinnamon Roasted Sweet Potato Chips

Ingredients (Serves 2)
- 1 medium sweet potato, peeled
- 2 tablespoons cold-pressed extra virgin coconut oil
- 2 teaspoons cinnamon
- Sea salt, to taste

Method
1. Preheat oven to 180°C.
2. Slice sweet potato into thin chip-like pieces.
3. Sprinkle with oil, cinnamon and salt and bake for 20 minutes.
4. Finish off under the grill until crispy.

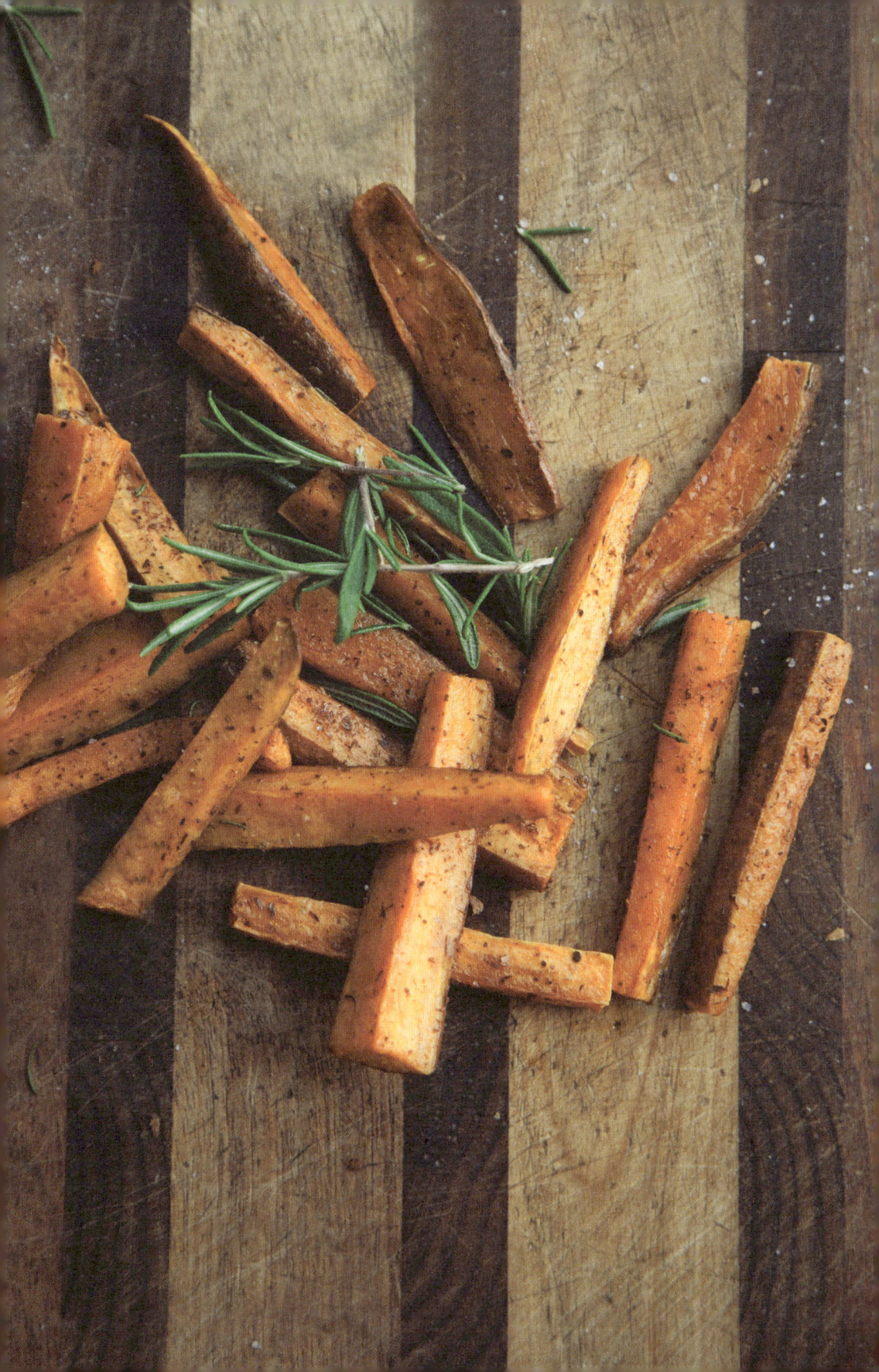

Roasted Vegies

Ingredients (Serves 4)
- 1 medium sweet potato, diced
- 1 beetroot, diced
- 1 zucchini, diced
- 1 garlic bulb, skinned and cloved
- 2 tablespoons cold-pressed extra virgin coconut oil
- 1-2 sprigs of fresh rosemary
- Sea salt, to taste

Method
1. Preheat oven to 180°C.
2. To a large baking tray, add chopped vegies.
3. Cover with coconut oil, rosemary and salt.
4. Cook for 20-30 minutes, turning once to ensure all slices are coated in oil and salt.
5. Remove from oven and allow to cool slightly.

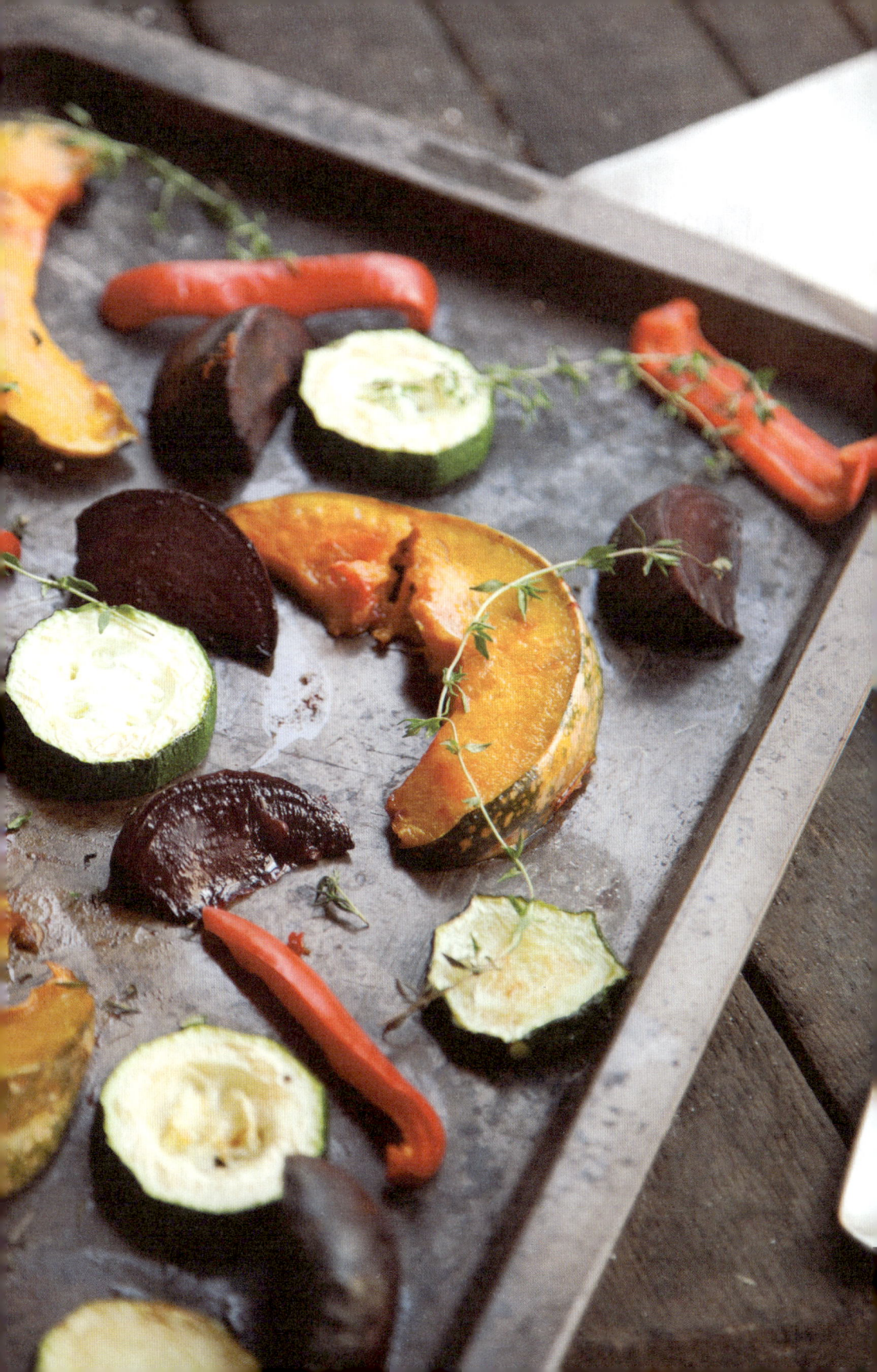

Pumpkin Mash

Ingredients (Serves 2-3)
- 1 medium pumpkin
- 2 tablespoons grass-fed butter
- Sea salt, to taste

Method
1. Remove skin and seeds and slice pumpkin into small pieces and steam until soft.
2. Mash with butter and season with salt to taste.

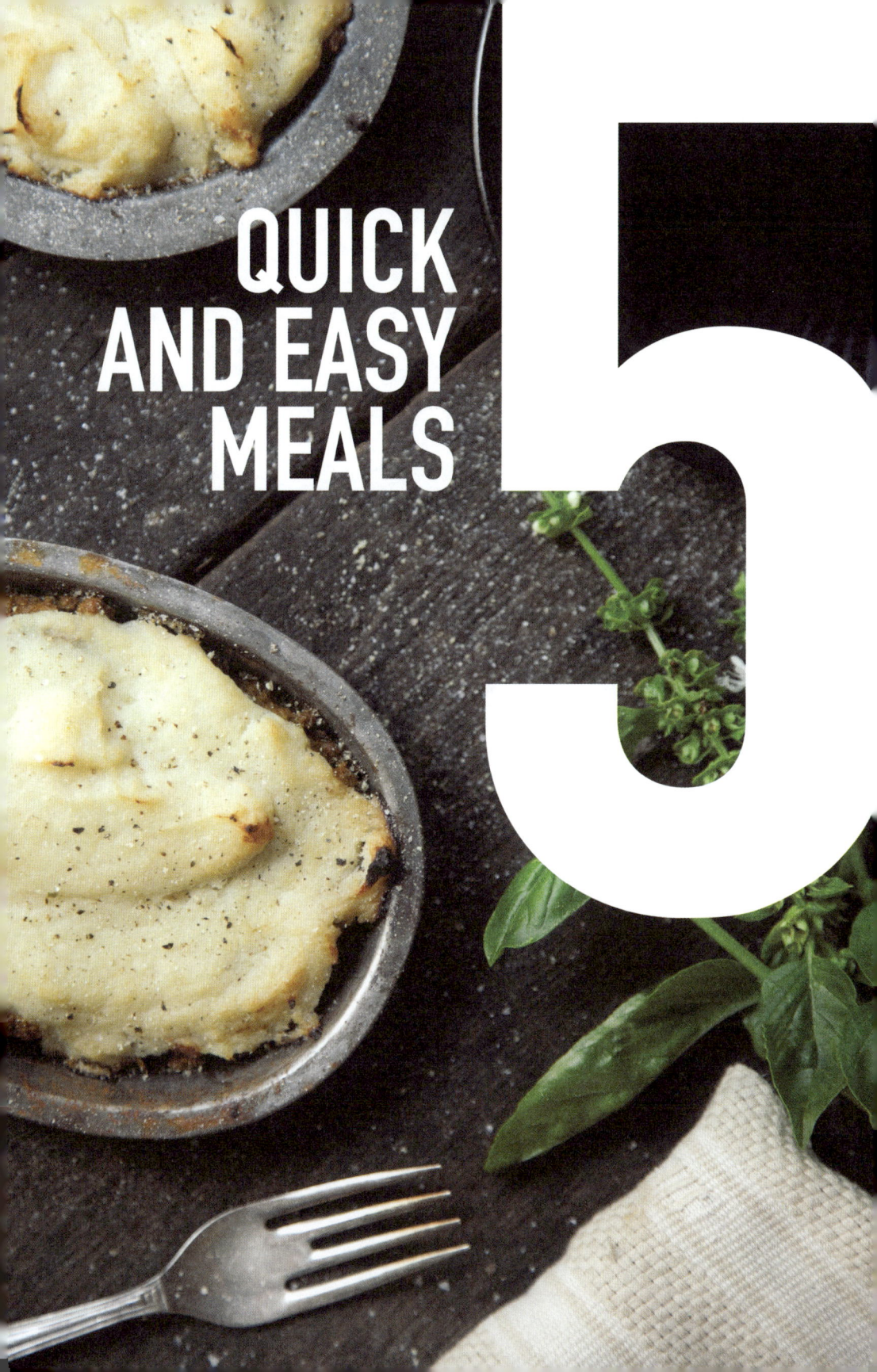

5
QUICK AND EASY MEALS

Grass-Fed Steak with Salad and Chips

Ingredients (Serves 2)
- 2 grass-fed steaks of your choice
- 1 teaspoon cold-pressed extra virgin coconut oil
- Sea salt and pepper, to taste
- Broccoli and Kale Salad (page 124)
- Cinnamon Roasted Sweet Potato Chips (page 148)

Method
1. Heat coconut oil in a pan and cook seasoned steak for 6-8 minutes on each side.
2. Remove from the heat, serve with Broccoli and Kale Salad and Cinnamon Roasted Sweet Potato Chips.

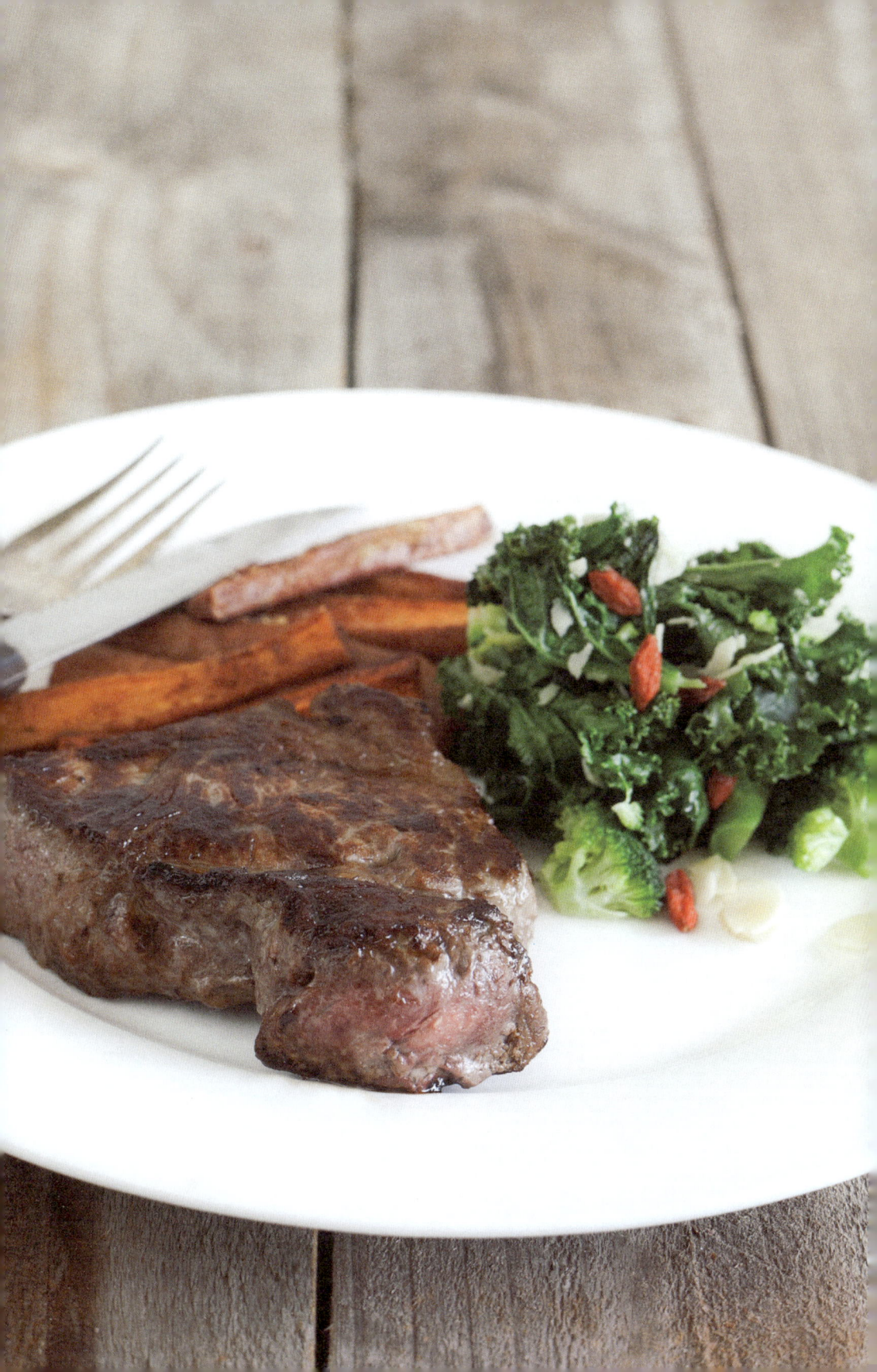

Clean Snags with Paleo Coleslaw

Ingredients (Serves 2)
- 1 tablespoon cold-pressed extra virgin coconut oil
- 4 grass-fed sausages
- 1 large carrot, grated
- 1/2 cabbage head, finely sliced
- Paleo Mayo (page 186)
- Sugar Free Tomato Sauce (page 182)

Method
1. Heat coconut oil in a pan and cook sausages for 6-8 minutes on each side.
2. To make coleslaw: add carrot, cabbage and Paleo Mayo to a large bowl and combine well.
3. Serve sausages topped with Sugar Free Tomato Sauce alongside coleslaw.

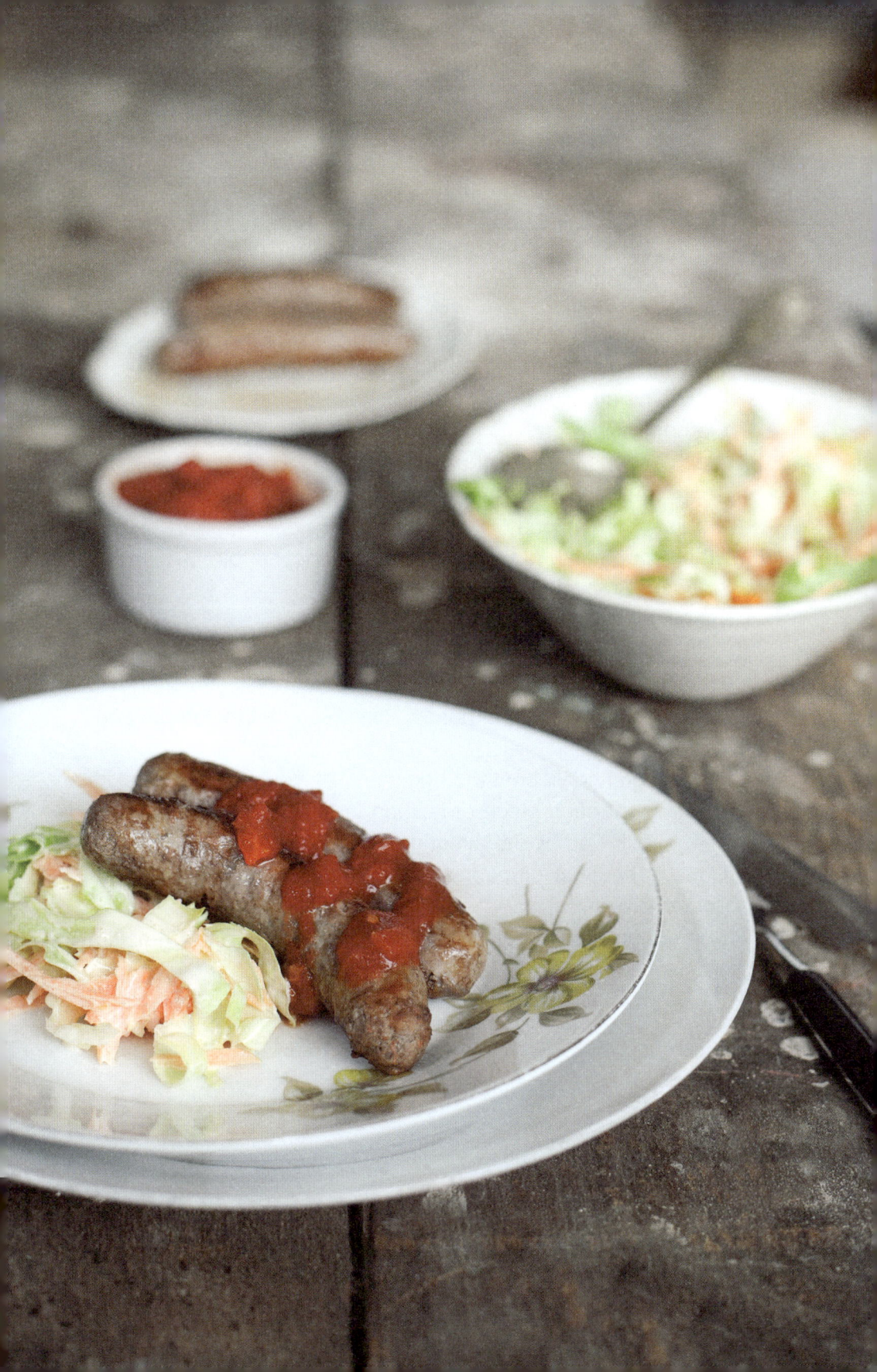

Almond Crusted Salmon with Greens and Mash

Ingredients (Serves 4)
- 4 salmon fillets, preferably wild-caught
- 1 cup almond flour or ground almonds
- 1 lemon
- 2 tablespoons parsley, chopped
- 1 egg, free range
- 1 tablespoon tapioca
- 1 tablespoon cold-pressed extra virgin coconut oil
- Steamed Broccolini with Feta (page 140)
- Pumpkin Mash (page 152)

Method
1. In a bowl, combine almonds, the zest of the lemon and parsley.
2. In a second bowl, beat the egg.
3. Lightly coat each piece of salmon in tapioca, before dipping in egg, followed by the almond mix.
4. Cook in coconut oil over a low to medium heat until lightly golden brown.
5. Serve alongside Steamed Broccolini with Feta and Pumpkin Mash.

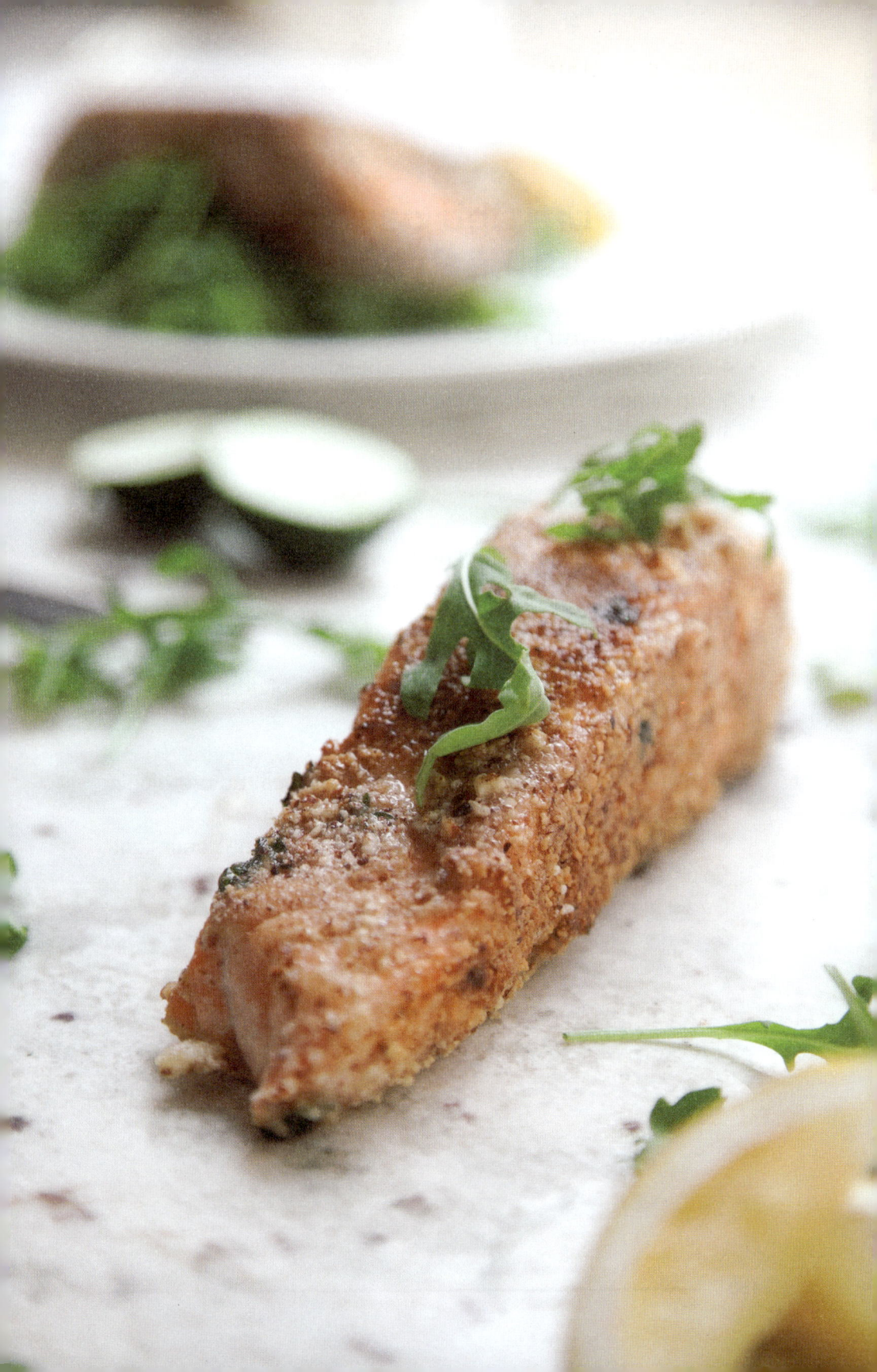

Gluten Free Chicken Schnitz with Broccolini Beauty

Ingredients (Serves 4)
- 4 chicken thigh, free range
- 1 cup almond flour or ground almonds
- 1 lemon
- 2 tablespoons parsley, chopped
- 1 egg, free range
- 1 tablespoon tapioca
- 1 tablespoon cold-pressed extra virgin coconut oil
- Broccolini Beauty (page 126)

Method
1. In a bowl, combine almonds, the zest of the lemon and parsley.
2. In a second bowl, beat the egg.
3. Lightly coat each piece of chicken in tapioca, before dipping in egg, followed by the almond mix.
4. Cook in coconut oil over a low to medium heat until lightly golden brown.
5. Serve alongside Broccolini Beauty.

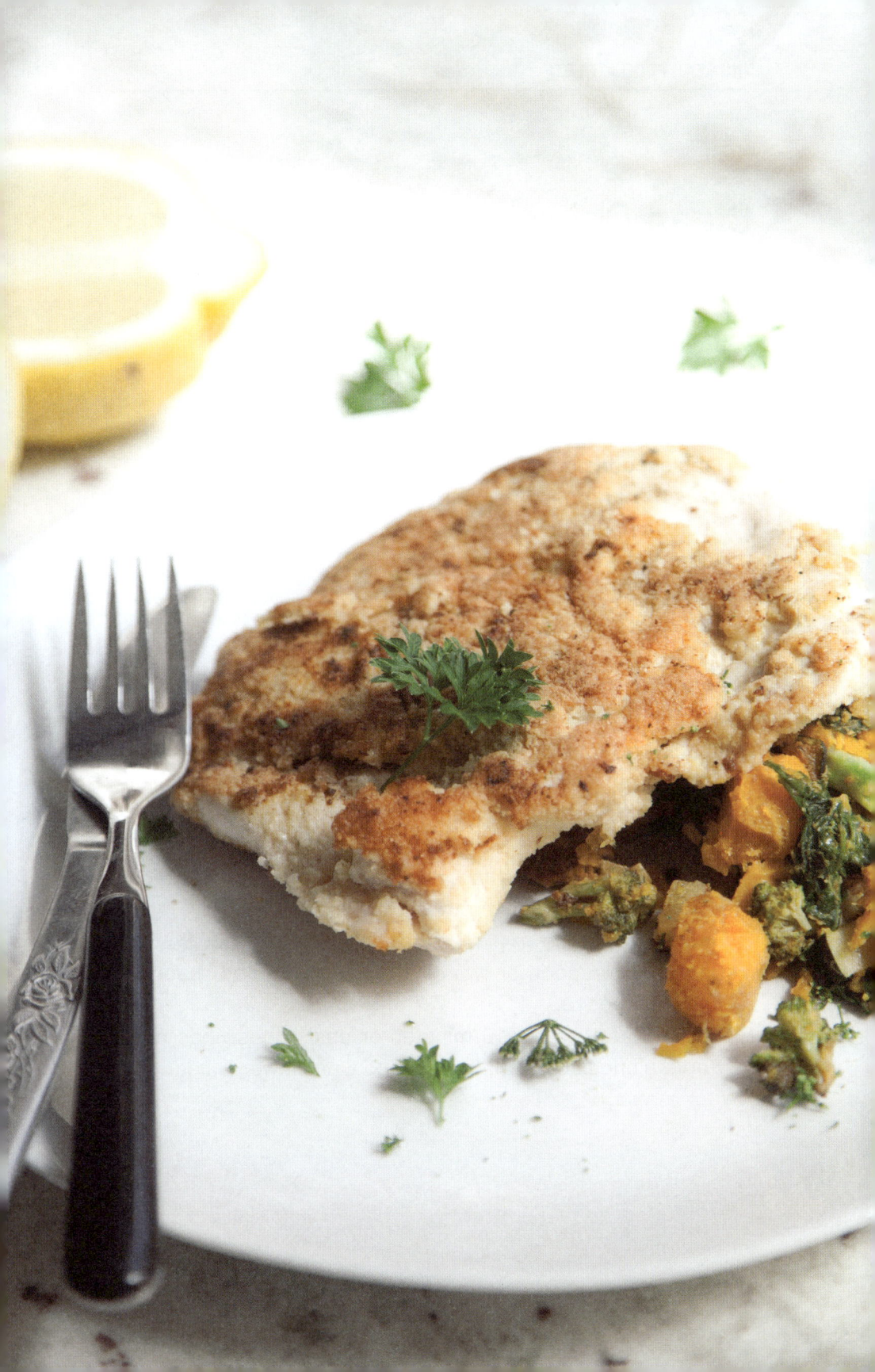

Clean Chicken Parma with Warm Fennel and Cauliflower Salad

Ingredients (Serves 2-3)
- 4 chicken thigh, free range
- 1 egg, free range
- 1 cup almond or hazelnut meal
- 1 tablespoon coconut flour
- 1/2 cup cold-pressed extra virgin coconut oil
- 4 pieces ham, free range
- Sugar Free Tomato Sauce (page 182)
- 8 slices organic hard cheese
- Warm Fennel and Cauliflower Salad (page 130)

Method
1. Pre-heat oven to 180°C.
2. Crack egg into a small bowl and whisk well. In a separate bowl, combine almond/hazelnut meal and coconut flour.
3. Cover chicken thighs well in egg, then coat well in the flour mix.
4. Heat coconut oil in a large pan and shallow fry chicken on both sides until lightly browned.
5. Transfer from the frypan onto a lined baking tray. Lay down ham, a tablespoon or two of Sugar Free Tomato Sauce and top with cheese.
6. Pop in the oven for 10 minutes or until cheese has melted. Serve alongside Warm Fennel and Cauliflower Salad.

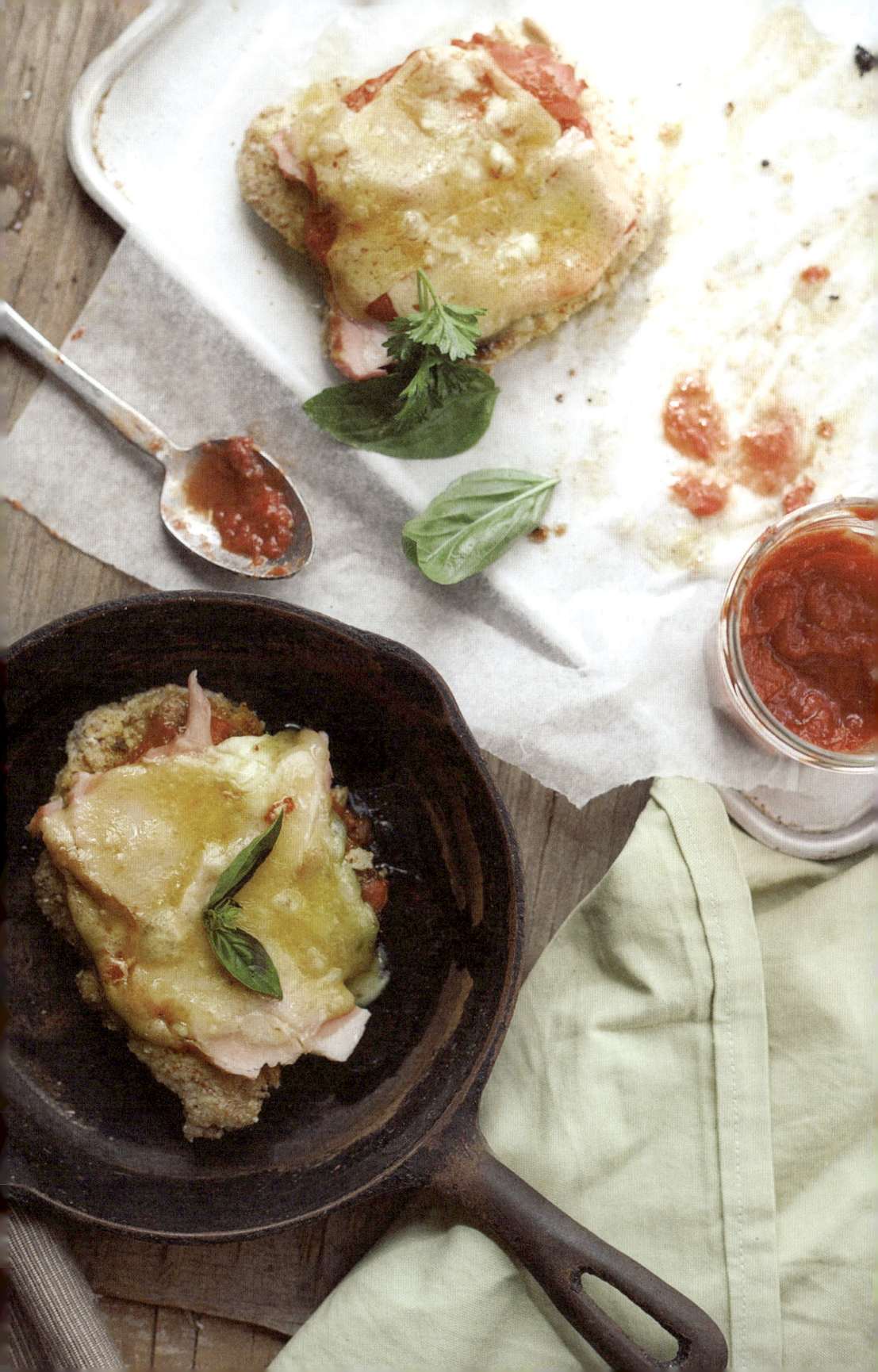

Shepherd's Pie with Cauliflower Mash

Ingredients (Serves 4-6)
- 1 tablespoon cold-pressed extra virgin coconut oil
- 2 garlic gloves, chopped
- 500g grass-fed beef mince
- 1 small can of anchovies, drained and chopped
- 400g tomato passata (100% tomatoes)
- 1 sachet tomato paste (no salt added)
- 1 teaspoon chilli flakes
- 1 teaspoon cinnamon
- 1 teaspoon nutmeg
- Sea salt, to taste
- Black pepper, to taste
- 3 celery stalks, chopped
- Cauliflower Mash (page 142)

Method
1. Preheat the oven to 220°C and heat the oil in a large pan. Sauté the garlic over a medium heat until golden brown.
2. Add the mince and anchovies and cook for 5 minutes, breaking up the meat.
3. Add the chopped tomatoes, tomato paste, herbs and spices and cook over a low heat until the excess liquid evaporates.
4. Add the celery to the mince mixture and transfer into an 18cm baking dish, spreading until level.
5. Gently spoon the mash over the top and press firmly until even.
6. Bake for 20 minutes and finish under the grill so the top is crispy and brown. Serve with your choice of salad.

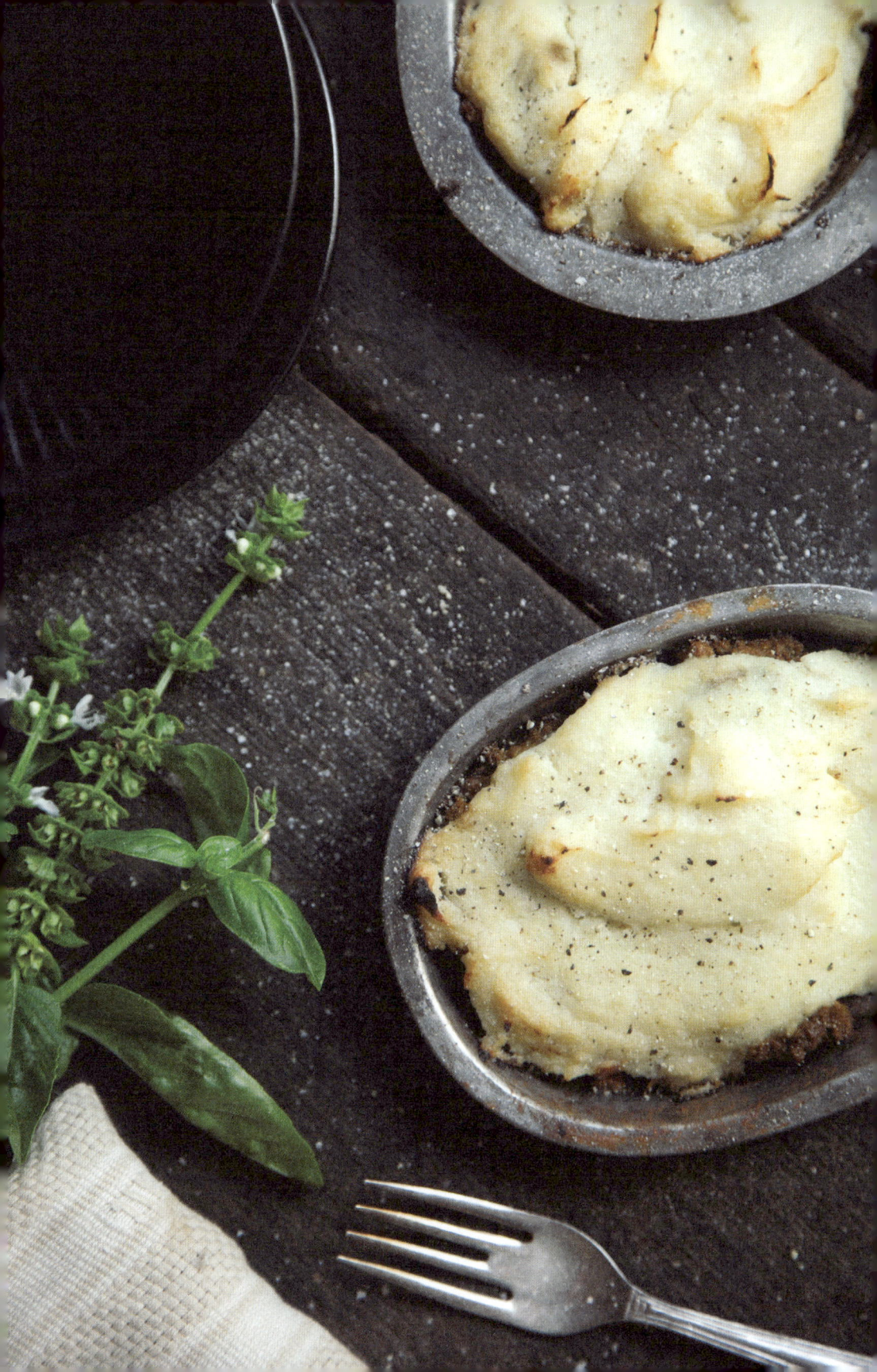

Zucchini Spaghetti Bolognese

Ingredients (Serves 2)
- 1 tablespoon cold-pressed extra virgin coconut oil
- 2 garlic gloves, finely chopped
- 200g grass-fed beef mince
- 400g tomato passata (100% tomatoes)
- 1 sachet tomato paste (no salt added)
- 1 teaspoon chilli flakes
- 1 teaspoon cinnamon
- 1 teaspoon nutmeg
- Sea salt, to taste
- Black pepper, to taste
- 2 zucchinis
- 1 carrot
- 1 tablespoon grass-fed butter
- 1 avocado, mashed

Method
1. Heat oil in a large pan and lightly brown garlic.
2. Add mince and brown lightly, stirring throughout.
3. Add tomatoes and tomato paste, herbs and spices. Simmer until most of liquid has evaporated. Set aside.
4. Grate 1 zucchini and carrot and stir through mince mixture.
5. Spiralise or slice the other zucchini to your desired thickness and serve raw or sauté in a saucepan with the butter.
6. Serve zucchini 'spaghetti' in a bowl, top with mince mixture and avocado.

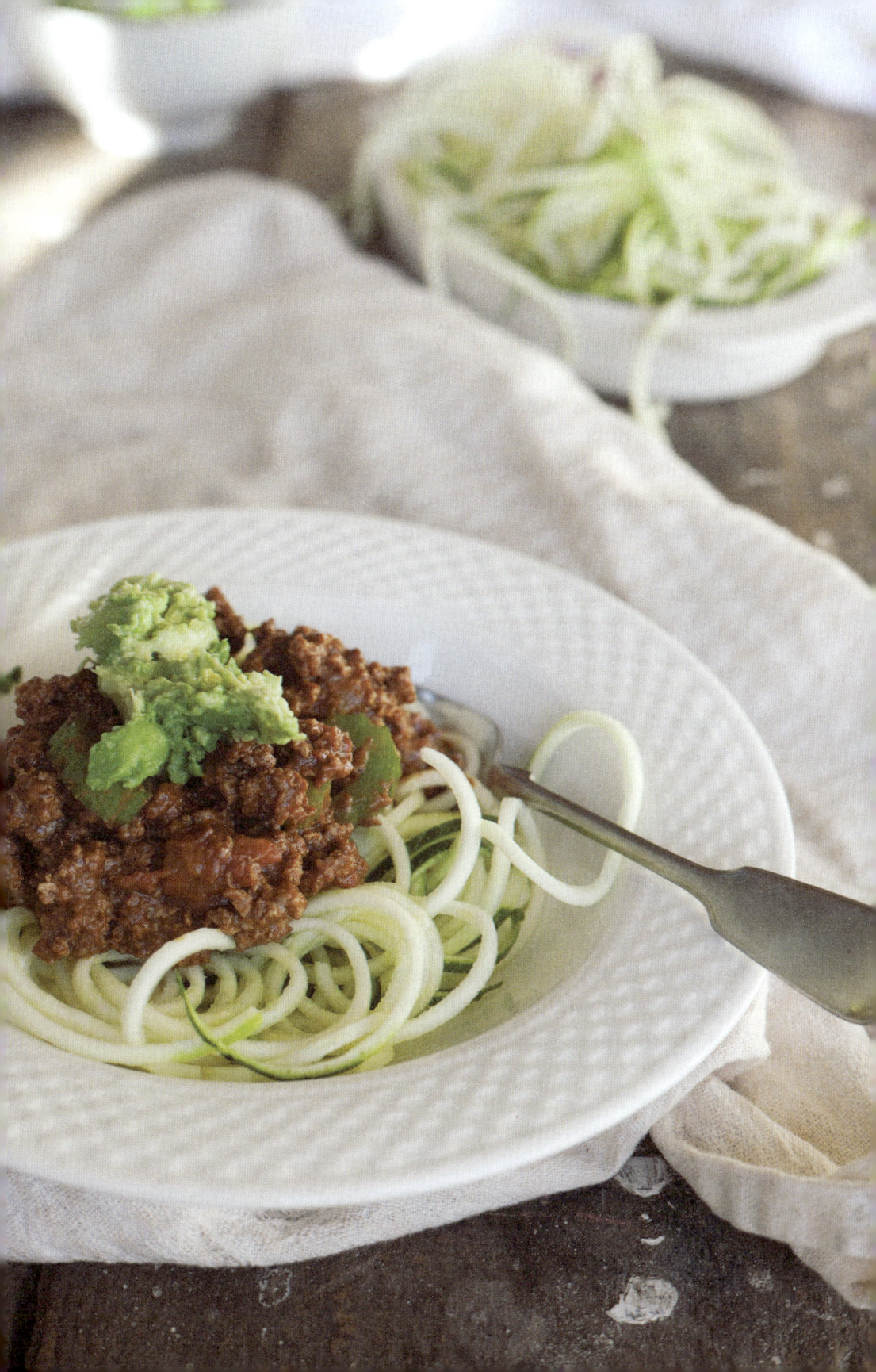

Green Chicken Curry with Cauliflower Rice

Ingredients (Serves 3-4)
- 2 green chillies
- 2 cloves garlic
- 1 stick lemongrass
- 1 tablespoon curry powder
- 1 tablespoon turmeric
- 1/4 cup cold-pressed extra virgin coconut oil, plus extra for cooking
- 1 400ml can coconut milk
- 1 400ml can coconut cream
- 1 small sweet potato, peeled and roughly chopped
- 500g free range chicken thigh, diced
- Sea salt and pepper, to taste
- 1 bunch brocollini
- 1 zucchini
- 1 cauliflower
- 1 lemon
- 1/4 bunch coriander

Method
1. Halve chillies and remove seeds. Roughly chop along with garlic and lemongrass and blend with curry powder, turmeric and coconut oil until a paste forms. If you are unfamiliar with lemongrass, simply remove the tough outer leaves and the bulb (end) and slice the stalk using all of the fleshy part. Stop slicing when you get to the greener, more woody section.
2. Heat 1 tablespoon oil in a large pan and cook paste for two minutes or until it becomes fragrant.

3. Add coconut milk, coconut cream, sweet potato and chicken and simmer for 15 minutes or until chicken is cooked and sweet potato is soft.
4. Season with salt and pepper to taste.
5. Add chopped, washed greens and simmer for 5 minutes.
6. Thoroughly wash cauliflower. De-stem, dice into small pieces and blitz in a food processor or blender until it resembles rice. Lightly sauté in coconut oil.
7. Serve curry on top of cauliflower rice with fresh coriander and a lemon wedge. Leftovers will keep in the fridge for 3-4 days.

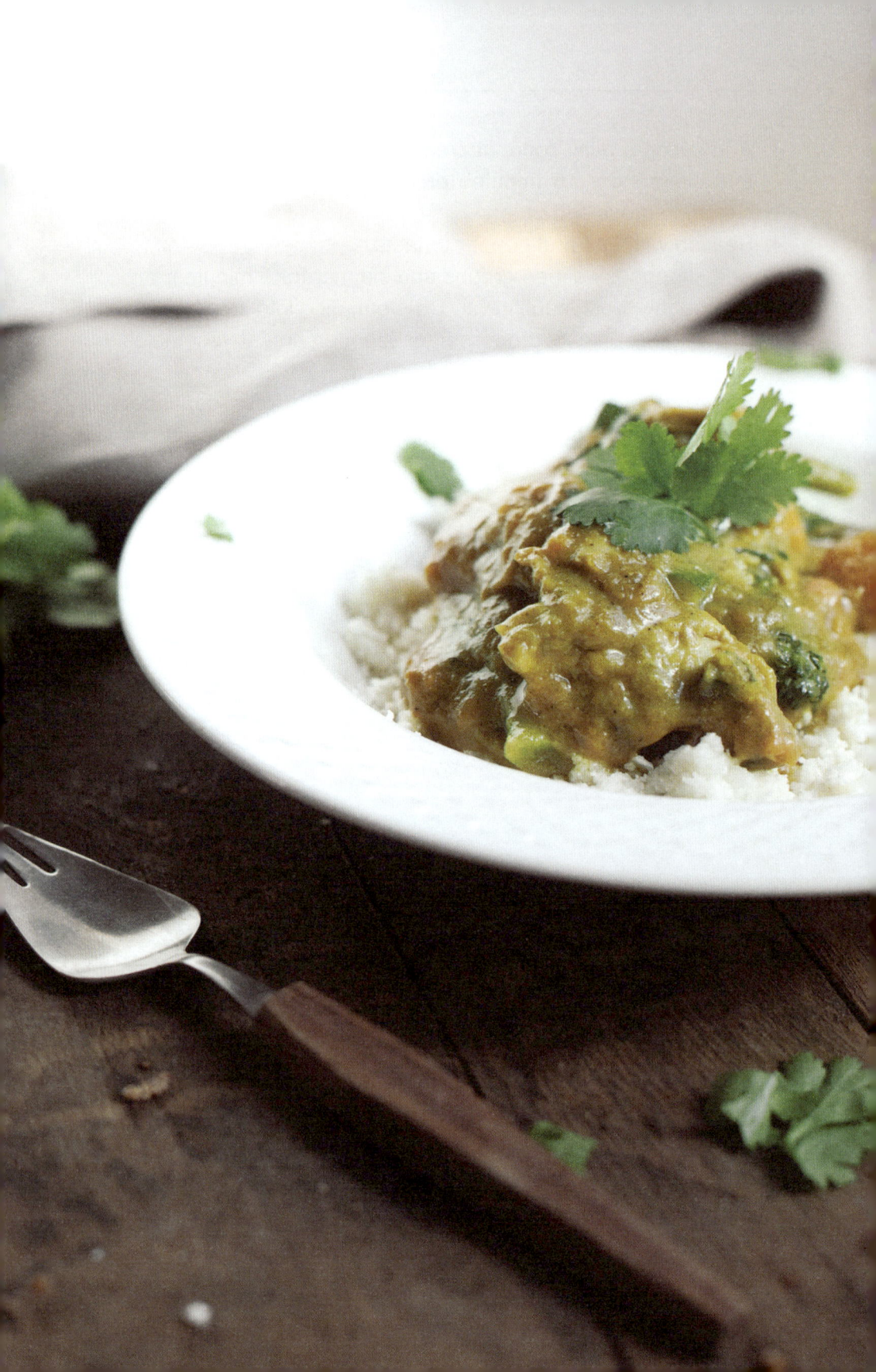

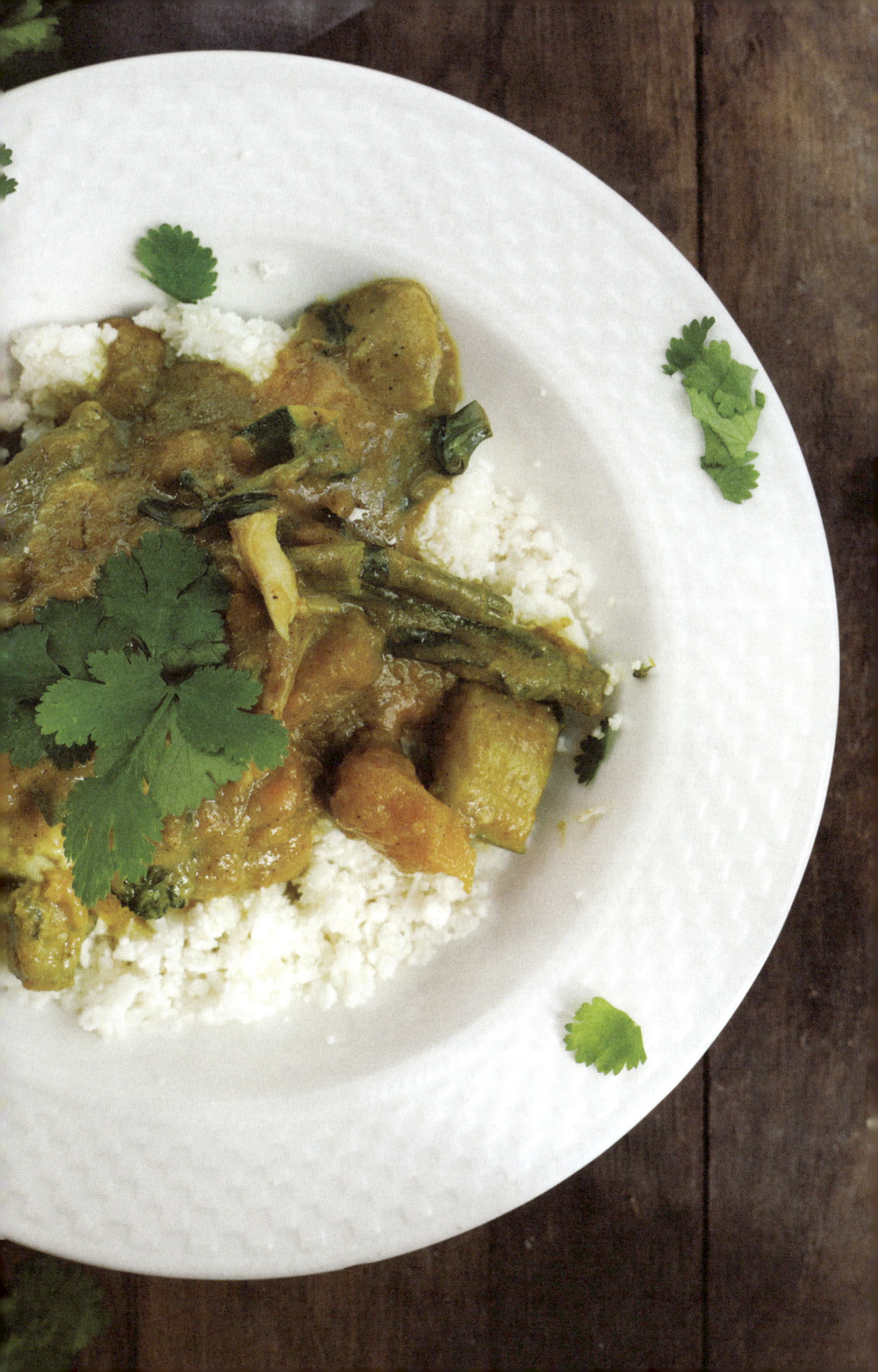

Clean Malaysian Fish Curry

Ingredients (Serves 3-4)
- 2 red chillies
- 2 cloves garlic
- 1 stick lemongrass
- 1 teaspoon curry powder
- 1 teaspoon turmeric
- 1/4 cup cold-pressed extra virgin coconut oil
- 1 400ml can coconut milk
- 1 400ml can coconut cream
- 1 small sweet potato, peeled and roughly chopped
- 2 fillets white fish
- 1 handful green beans
- 1 zucchini

Method
1. Halve chillies and remove seeds. Roughly chop along with garlic and lemongrass and blend with curry powder, turmeric and coconut oil until a paste forms. If you are unfamiliar with lemongrass, simply remove the tough outer leaves and the bulb (end) and slice the stalk using all of the fleshy part. Stop slicing when you get to the greener, more woody section.
2. Heat 1 tablespoon oil in a large pan and cook paste for two minutes or until it becomes fragrant.
3. Add coconut milk, coconut cream and sweet potato and simmer for 15 minutes or until sweet potato is soft.
4. Add the fish once the sweet potato is cooked and simmer for 5-10 minutes.
5. Finally, add chopped greens and simmer for 5 minutes.
6. Serve on top of cauliflower rice or cooked quinoa.

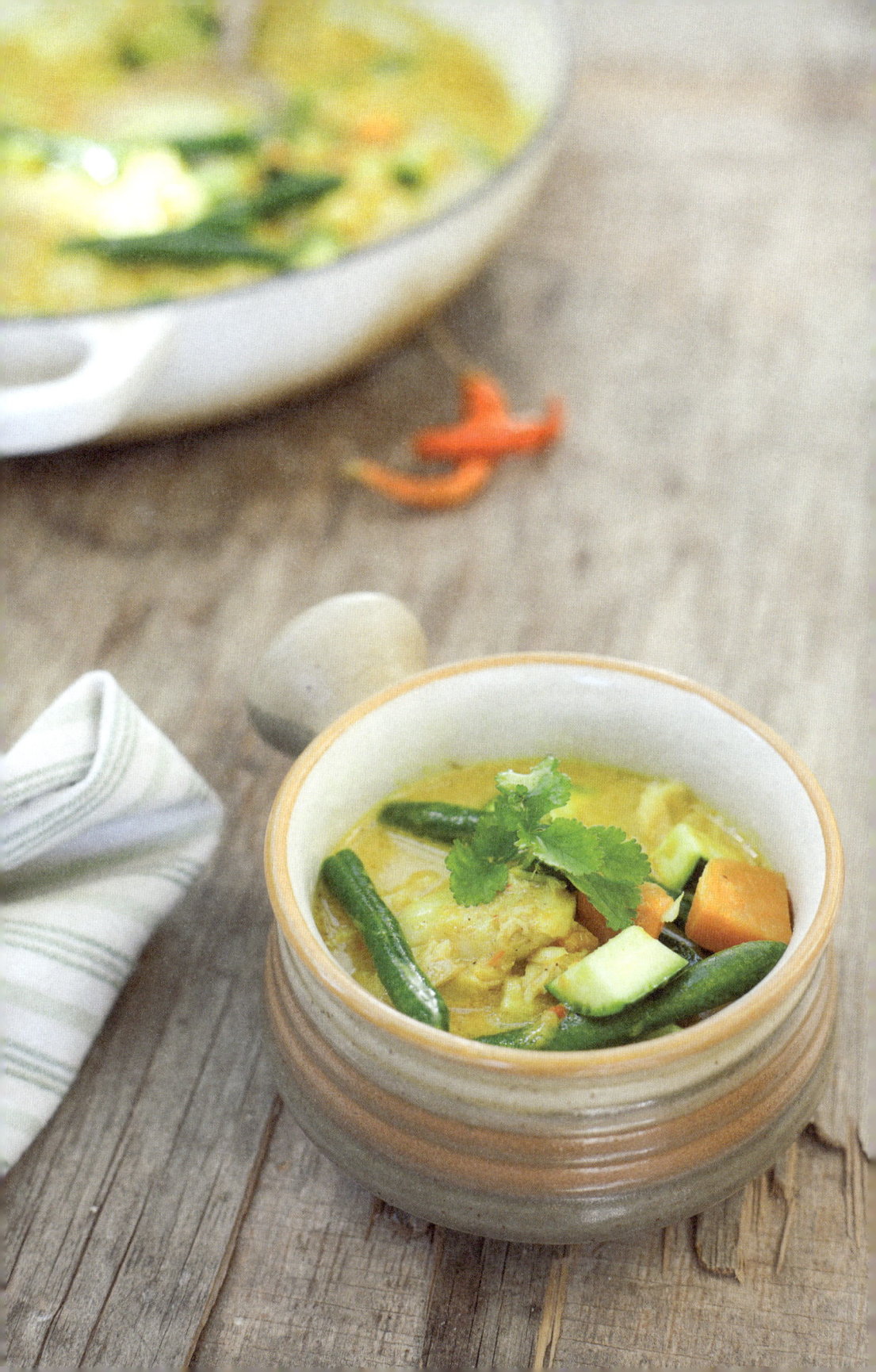

Paleo Quiche

Ingredients (Serves 4-6)

Base:
- 1 1/2 cups almond meal
- 1/2 cup coconut flour
- 1 teaspoon gluten free baking powder
- 1/2 teaspoon sea salt
- 2 eggs, free range
- 1/4 cup cold-pressed extra virgin coconut oil

Filling:
- 6 eggs, free range
- 1 handful semi sundried tomatoes, finely chopped
- 1 handful spinach, finely chopped
- 1 small handful pine nuts
- Sea salt, to taste
- Freshly ground pepper, to taste

Method
1. Preheat oven to 180°C.
2. To make the base, combine the flours with the baking powder and salt.
3. Beat and add the eggs and the stir through the oil.
4. Combine the mixture thoroughly with your hands and carefully press into a lightly greased quiche pan.
5. Cook for 10 minutes or until lightly golden.
6. To make the filling, beat the eggs and stir through the vegetables and pine nuts.
7. Season with salt and pepper and pour onto the lightly cooked base.
8. Cook for another 10 minutes or until firm to touch.
9. Cool before slicing and serving. Serve with your choice of salad.

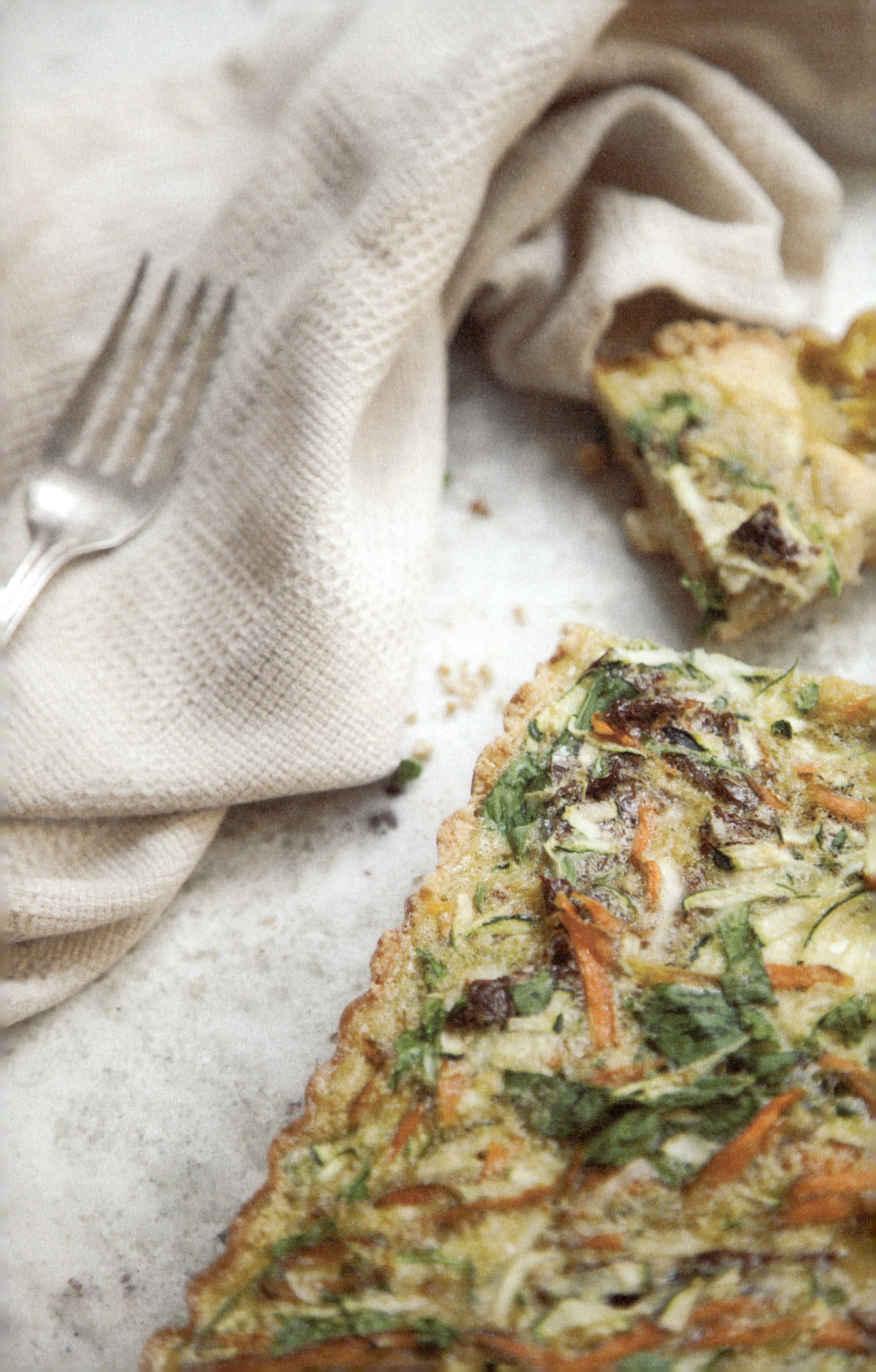

Grain Free Burger Bun

Ingredients (Serves 1)
- 2 eggs, free range
- 2 tablespoons almond flour
- 2-3 tablespoons coconut flour
- 1 tablespoon cold-pressed extra virgin coconut oil
- 1 teaspoon gluten free baking powder
- 1 teaspoon tapioca
- 1/2 teaspoon psyllium
- 1/2 teaspoon sea salt

Method
1. Preheat oven to 180C.
2. To make the bun, whisk eggs and combine well in a large bowl with all other ingredients. Add a touch more coconut flour if your mixture is too wet.
3. Split mixture into two and spoon into patty sized mounds on a baking tray lined with grease-proof paper. Spread evenly with the back of a spoon to create the shape and size you desire.
4. Cook for 15-20 minutes or until golden brown, flipping halfway.
5. Serve with your favourite fillings, such as a beef patty, sliced tomato, avocado, a fried egg and Sugar Free Tomato Sauce.

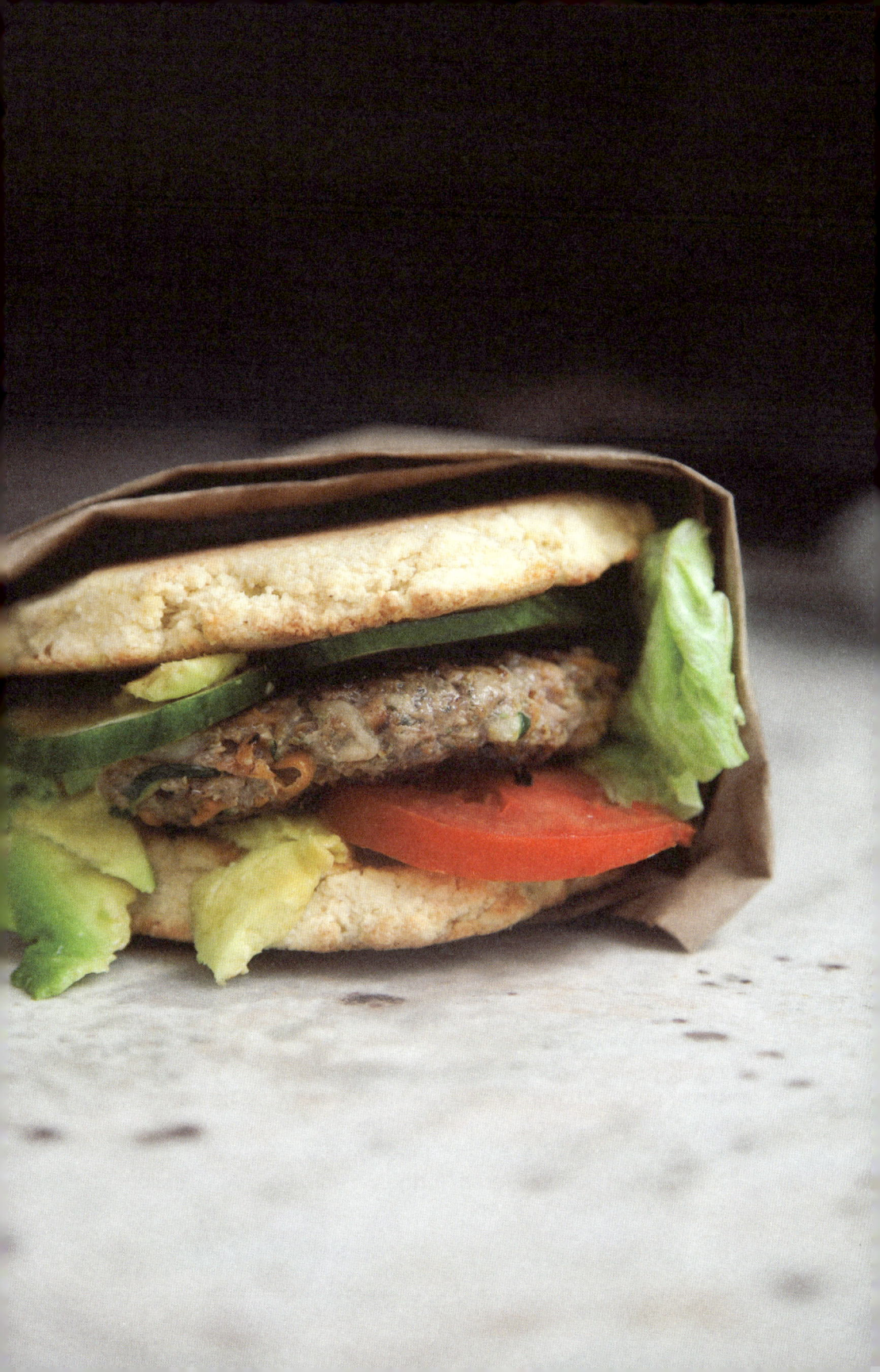

Cauliflower Pizza

Ingredients (Serves 2)
- 1/2 small cauliflower
- 1 cup almond meal
- 1/4 cup coconut flour
- 1 tablespoon tapioca
- 2 tablespoons psyllium husks
- 2 teaspoon gluten free baking powder
- 1/4 teaspoon sea salt
- 1 egg, free range
- 1/4 cup grass-fed butter
- 2 tablespoons Sugar Free Tomato Sauce (page 182)
- Toppings of your choice
- Cashew Cheese, optional (page 188)

Method
1. Preheat oven to 200°C.
2. Chop the cauliflower into florets and steam until very soft. Mash or blend until fine and set aside.
3. Add the almond meal, coconut flour, tapioca, psyllium, baking powder and salt to a large bowl and mix well.
4. Beat the egg and melt the butter and add both to the above mixture.
5. Add the cauliflower and stir thoroughly. Let this sit for a minute so all of the moisture from the cauliflower is absorbed.
6. Pour the mixture into a lightly greased quiche tin or onto a pizza tray. Use a bit of love here to spread the base evenly and firmly press down with your hands. To prevent sticking, lightly grease your hands first.
7. Cook for 25-30 minutes or until lightly brown. The longer you leave it here, the crunchier it will be.
8. Evenly spread the Sugar Free Tomato Sauce, add your toppings and cook for a further 5 minutes. Add dollop of cashew cheese and serve.

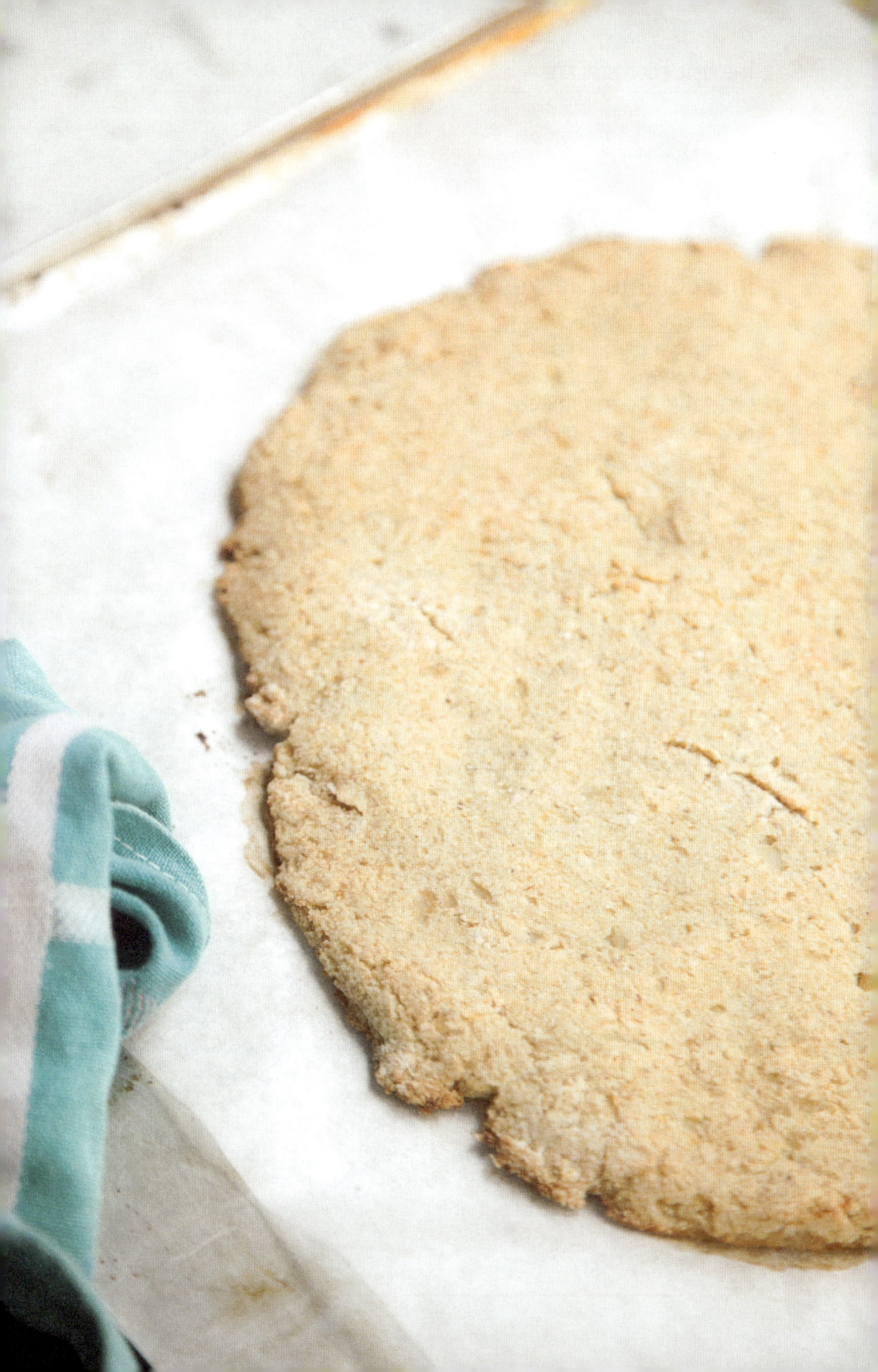

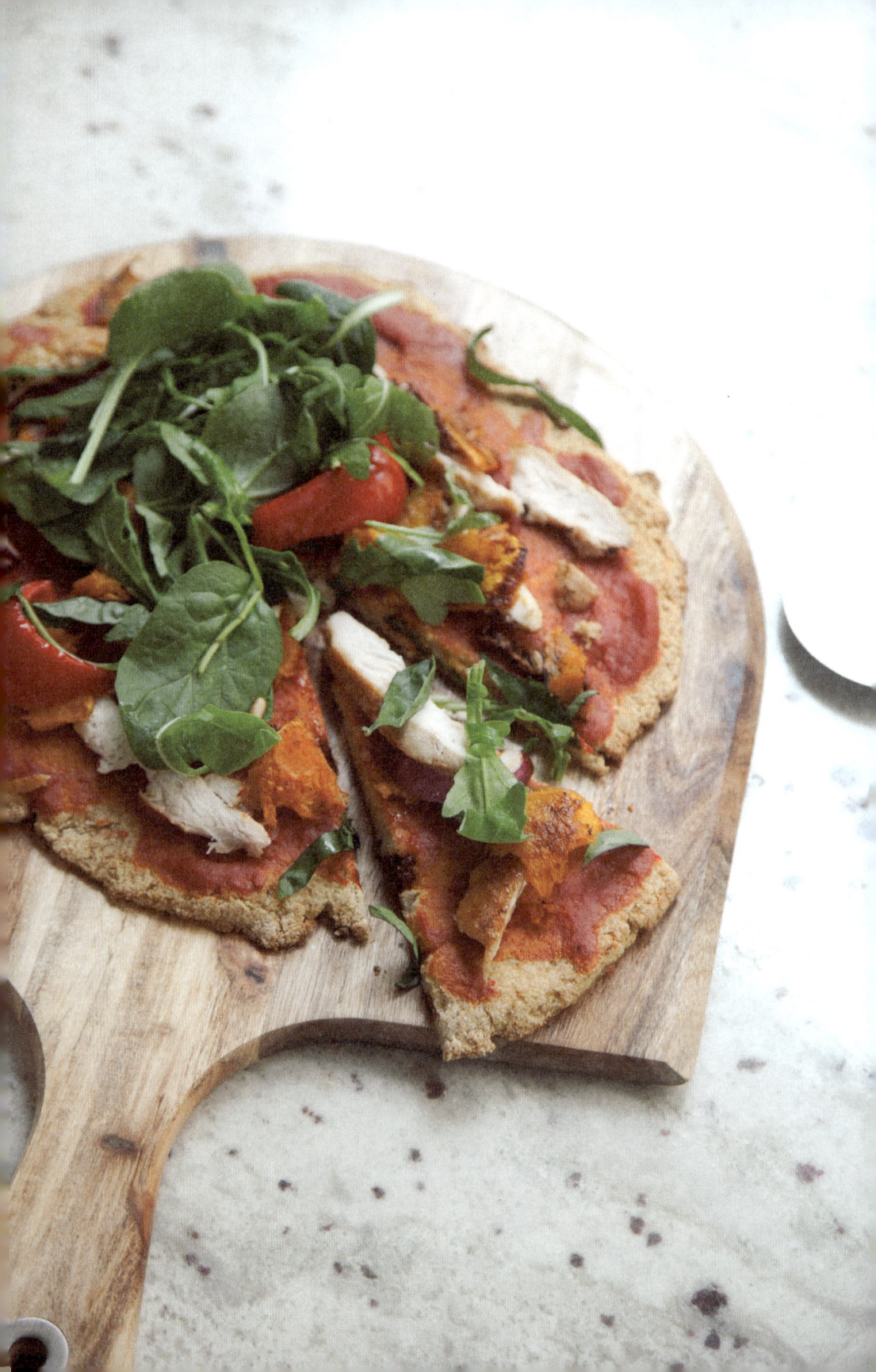

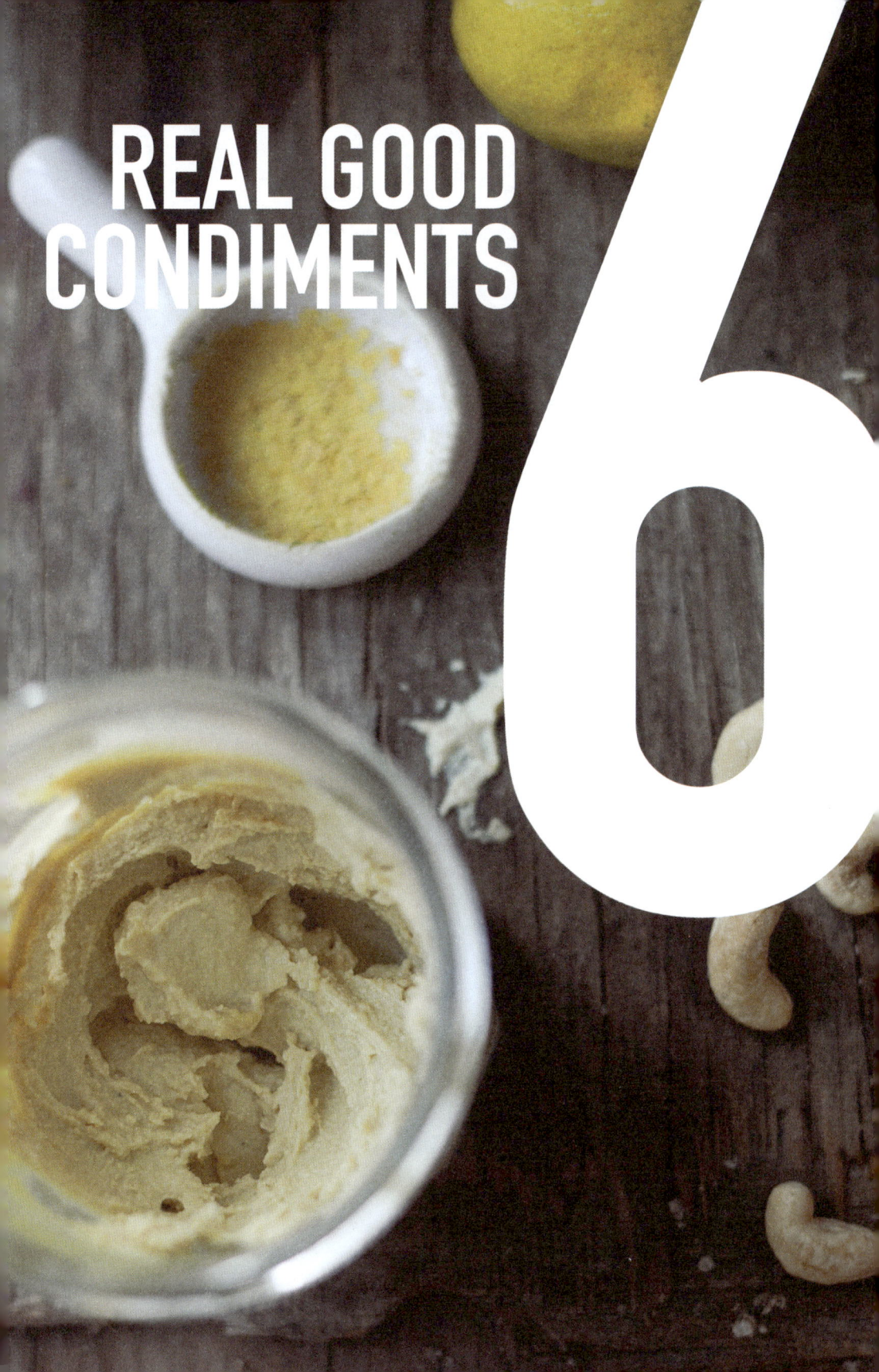

REAL GOOD CONDIMENTS

6

Sugar Free Tomato Sauce

Ingredients
- 1 teaspoon cold-pressed extra virgin coconut oil
- 1 garlic clove, finely chopped or crushed
- 400g tomato passata (100% tomatoes)
- 1 sachet tomato paste (no salt added)
- 1/2 cup apple cider vinegar (ACV)
- 1/4 tablespoon sea salt
- 1 tablespoon Pure Harvest organic rice malt syrup

Method
1. In a large pan, brown garlic in coconut oil over a medium heat.
2. Add all other ingredients and bring to the boil.
3. Reduce the heat and simmer until thick.
4. Cool and store in the fridge for up to three weeks.

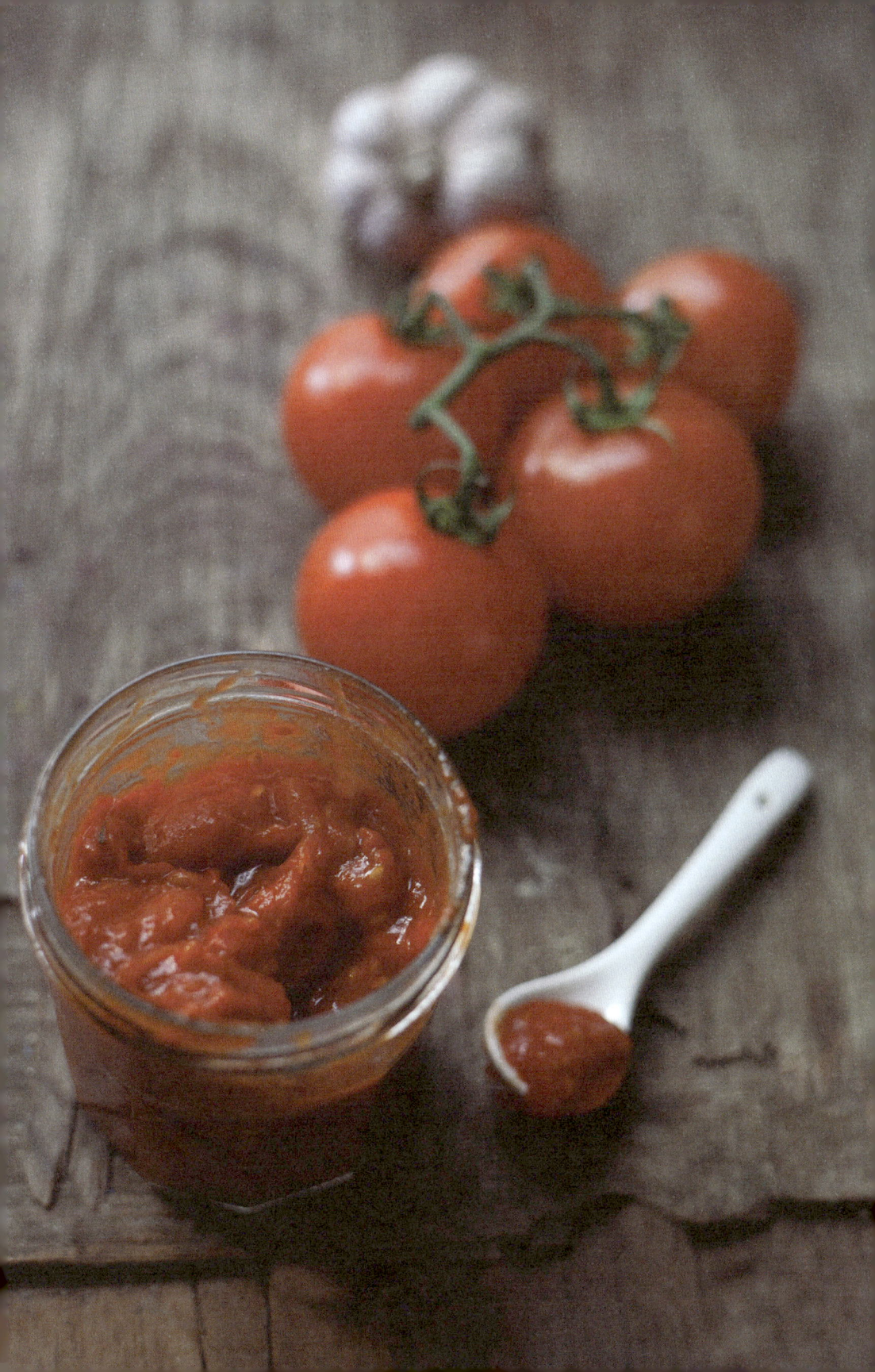

Cashew Sour Cream

Ingredients
- 1 cup soaked cashews
- 1/2 cup water
- 1/4 cup extra virgin olive oil (EVOO)
- The juice of one lemon
- Sea salt, to taste

Method
1. Combine all ingredients in a food processor or high-speed blender and process until smooth.
2. Transfer into a jar and store the fridge for up to a week.

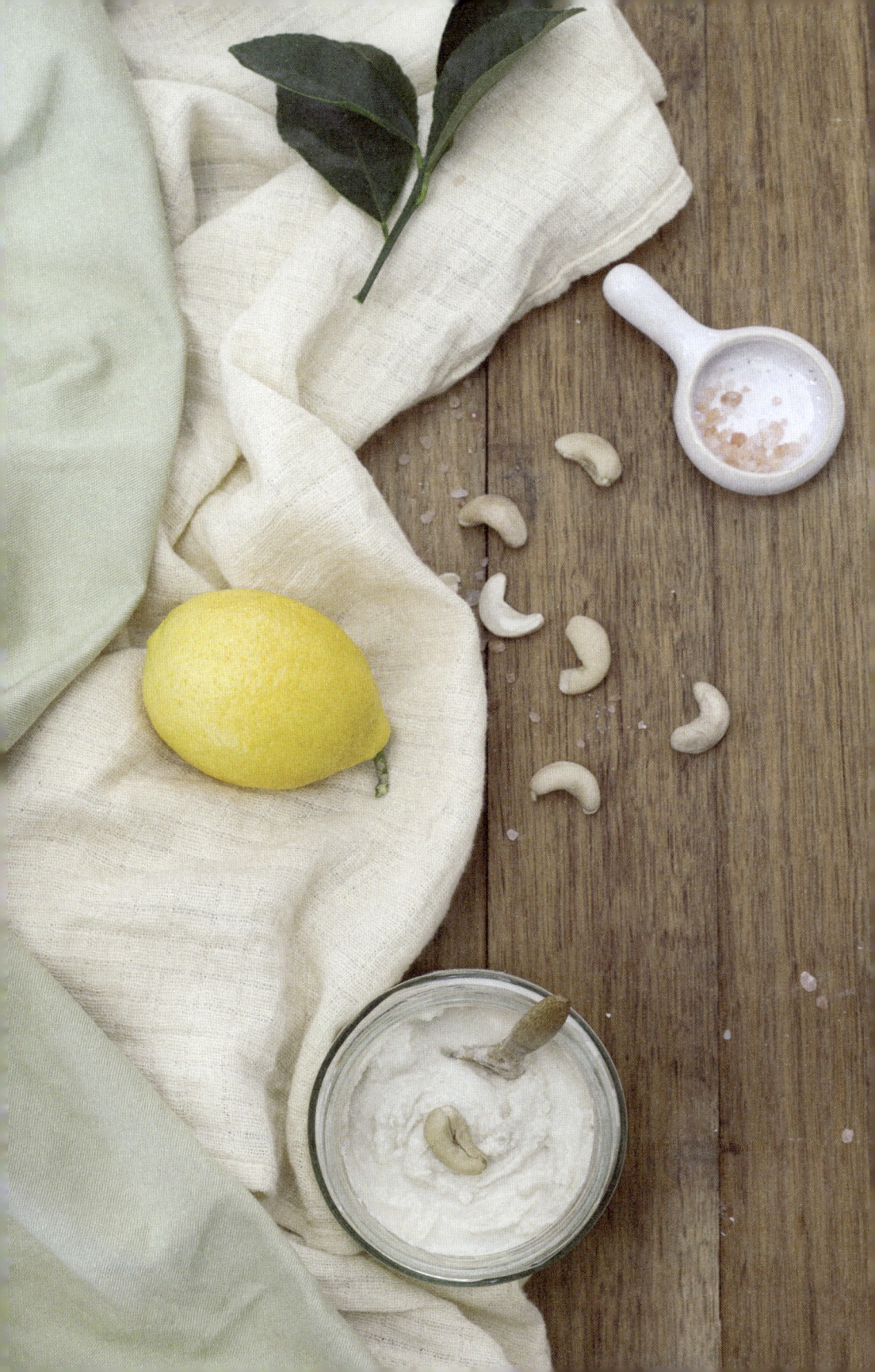

Paleo Mayo

Ingredients
- 1 large egg, free range
- 1 tablespoon lemon juice
- 1 tablespoon apple cider vinegar (ACV)
- 1 teaspoon mustard powder
- 3/4 cup macadamia/extra virgin olive oil (EVOO)
- 1/4 teaspoon sea salt

Method
1. In a blender or food processor, blend egg, lemon juice, ACV and mustard powder.
2. Slowly* add in oil, one tablespoon at a time, continuing to blend.
3. Add the salt once a creamy mayo has formed.
4. Transfer into a jar and store up until the used by date on your carton of eggs.

*The secret to this mayo is patience. Otherwise, it will split and you will be left with liquid, rather than a thick creamy blend. If your mayo does split, the good news is you can save it. Pour the liquid into a jar and place it in the coldest part of your fridge. Wait a few hours then blend again or beat vigorously with an egg beater. It will be slightly less thick and creamy than it should be, but still delicious and useful for salads.

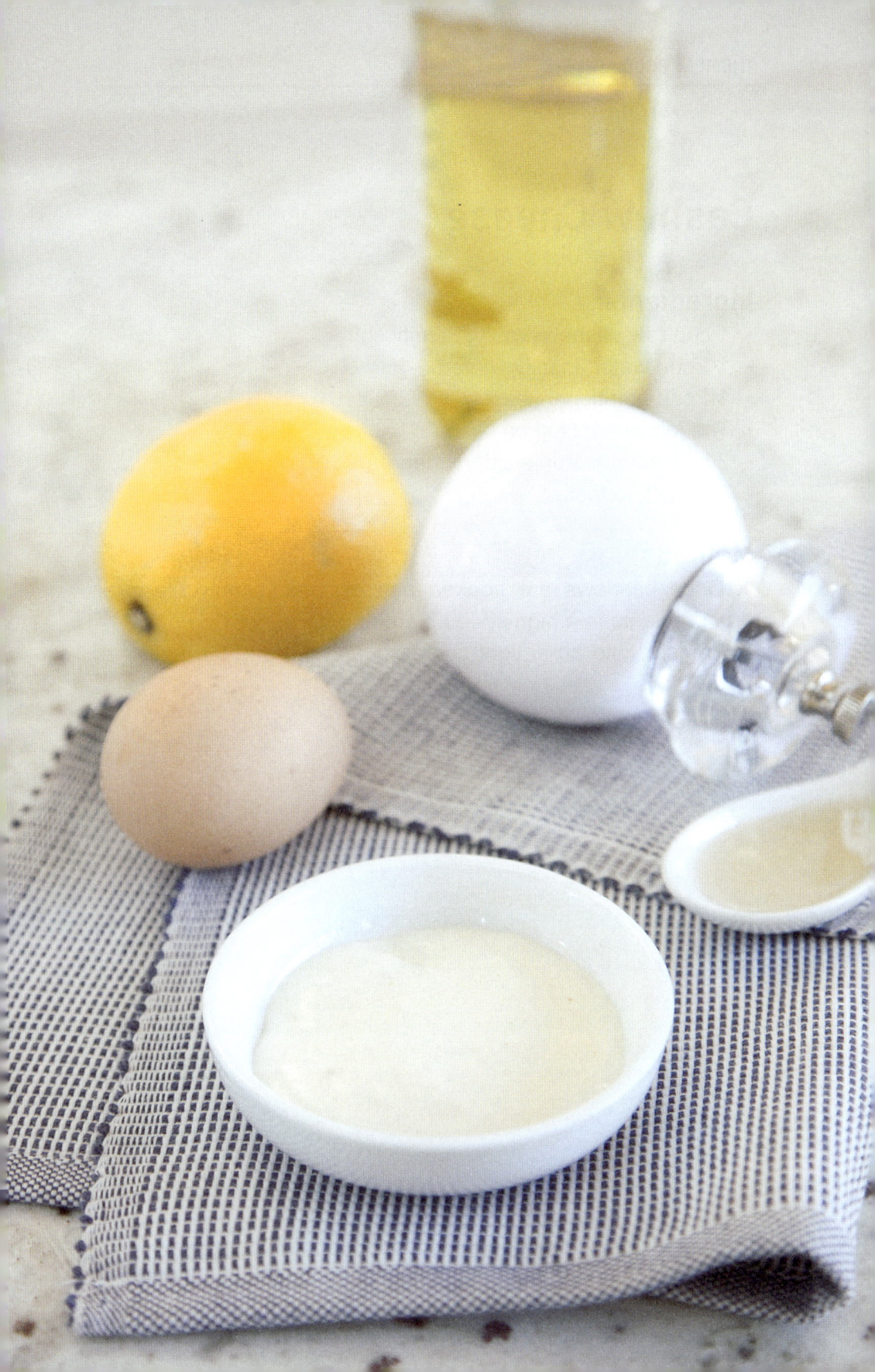

Cashew Cheese

Ingredients
- 1 cup raw cashews, soaked until soft
- 1/4 cup water, ideally filtered
- 1/4 cup nutritional yeast
- The juice of 1/2 lemon
- 2 tablespoons apple cider vinegar (ACV)
- Sea salt, to taste

Method
1. Once cashews are soaked and drained, simply blend all ingredients in a high-speed blender until smooth.
2. Transfer into an airtight container and store in the fridge for 5-7 days.

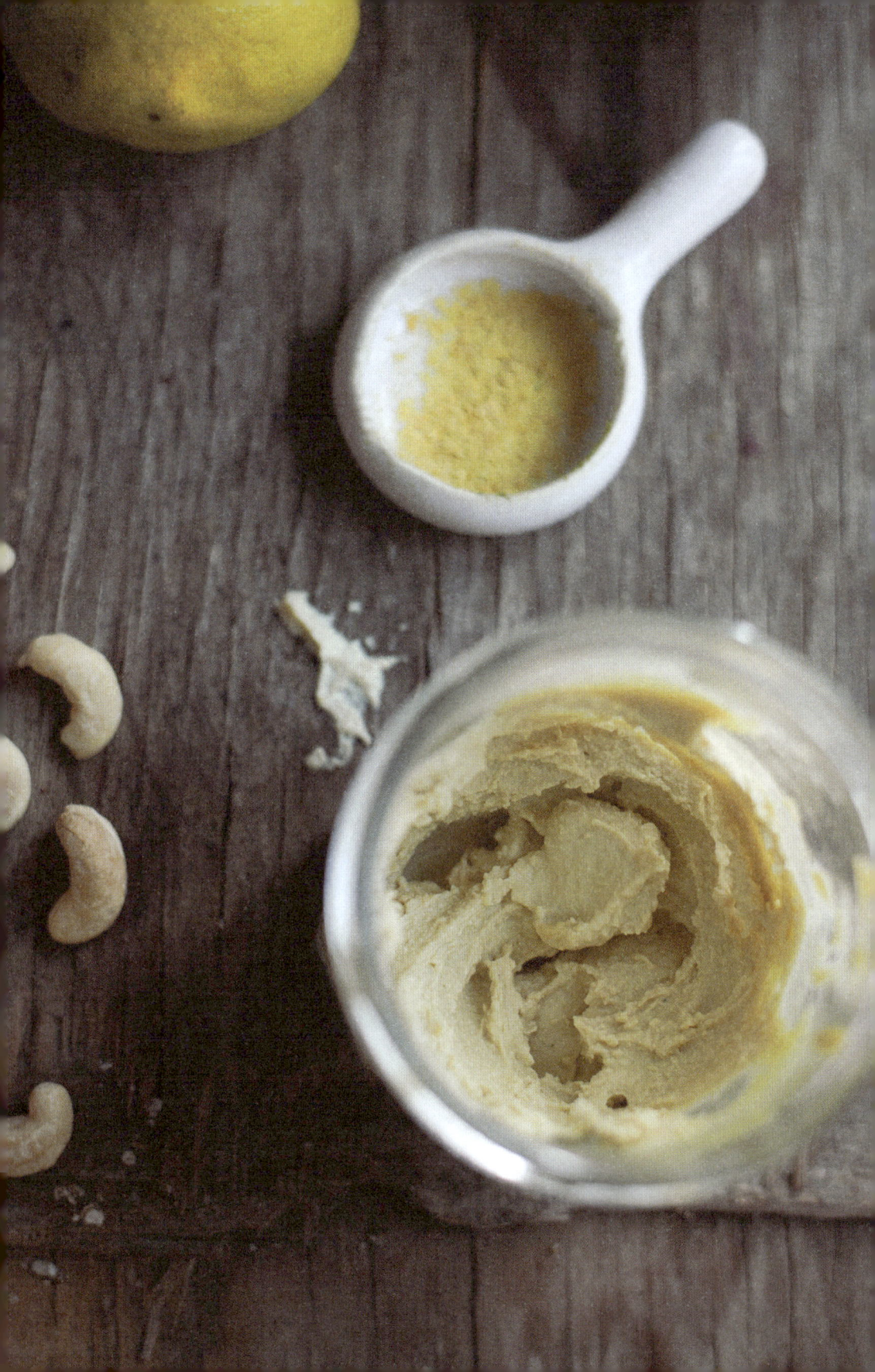

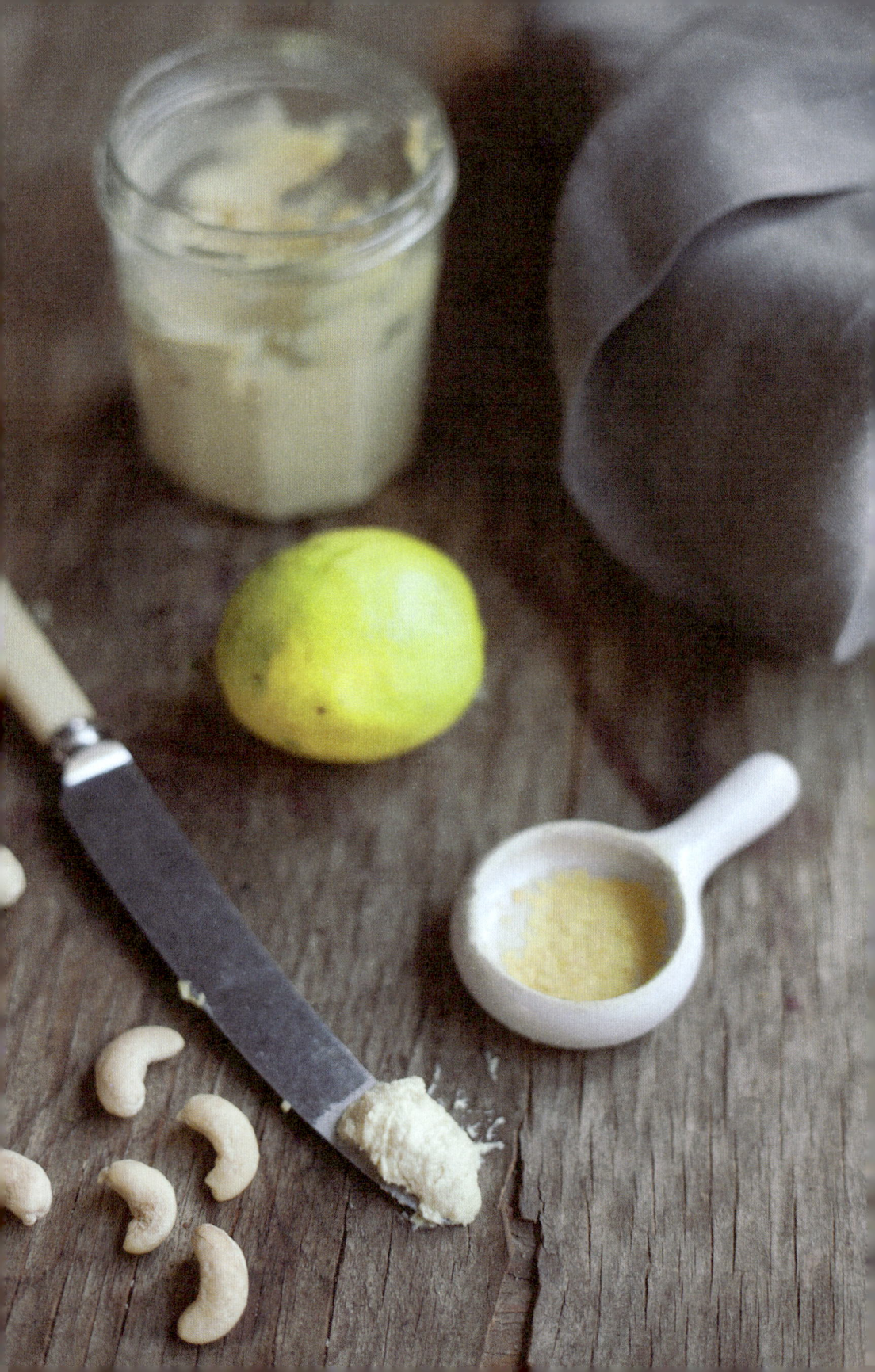

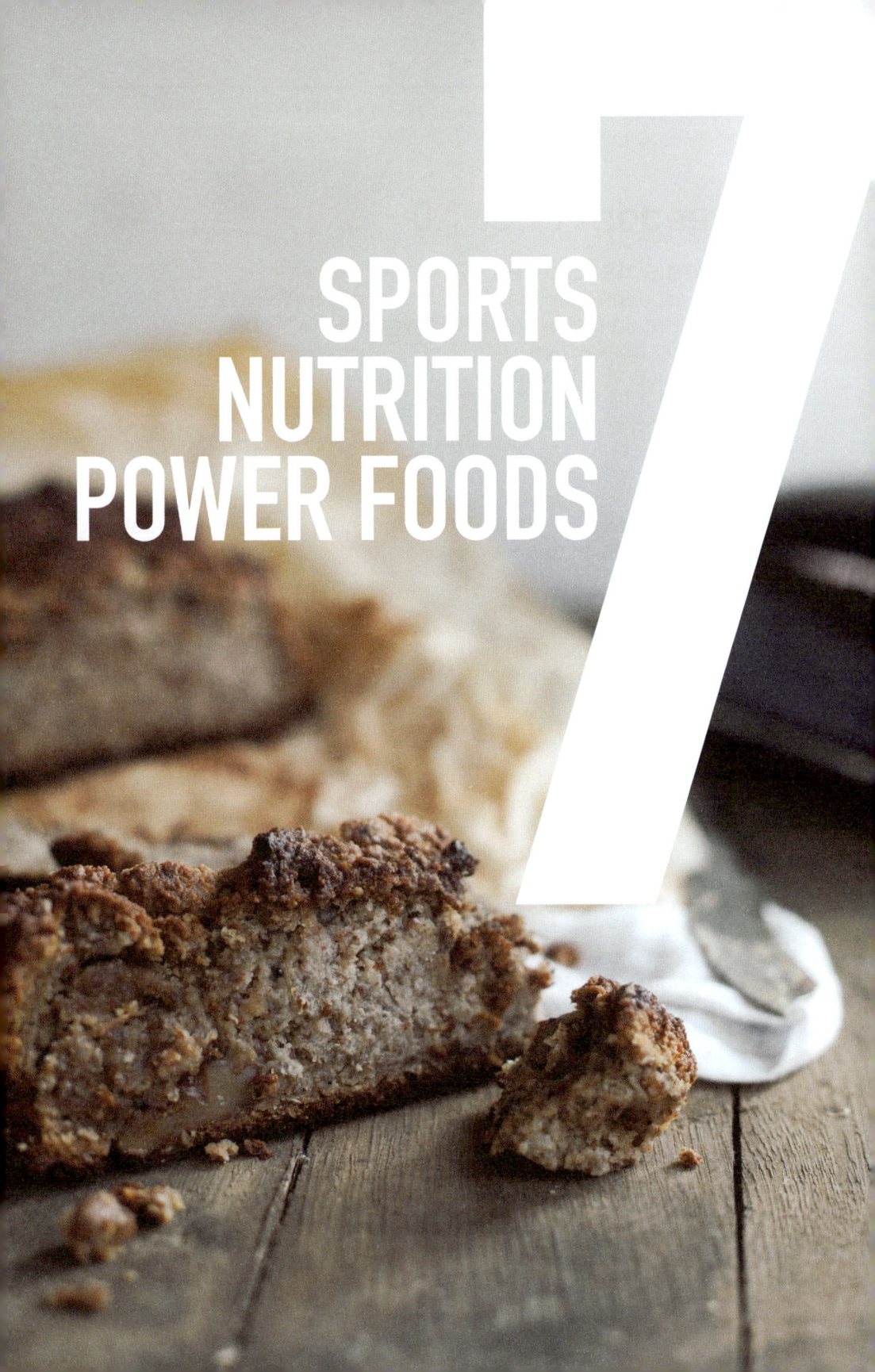

7 SPORTS NUTRITION POWER FOODS

Freedom Fuel 1.0

Ingredients (Serves 1)
- 2 teaspoons Pure Harvest organic rice malt syrup
- 1 teaspoon medium chain triglyceride (MCT) oil
- 1/4 cup raspberries
- The juice of 1/4 lemon
- A pinch of sea salt
- A dash of hot water

Method
1. Blend all ingredients until smooth.
2. Pour through a strainer to remove pips. Transfer carefully into a gel flask and seal well.

Notes
1. Coconut oil is fine in warmer weather but it will solidify and clog the pop-top of your flask/bottle in cooler weather, so MCT oil is preferable here.
2. For MCT oil, a brand such as Melrose is available here: bit.ly/tnnonline
3. Blueberries or strawberries can be used in place of raspberries.
4. Once made, it will only last for two days but freezes well.
5. If you are training/racing in warmer weather please consider freezing your FF.
6. FF may not be suitable for 'special needs' during a hot race as it is possible that the fruit may start to ferment. In this situation we recommend VFuel, available here: bit.ly/tnnonline
7. One serve is ~20g of carbohydrates, so please start to experiment with 30-40g/hour or 1.5-2.0 serves/hour. For a two hour run, for example, train fasted for the first hour, then sip your 1.5 serves over the course of the second hour. Make notes of energy, digestion, performance and recovery so we can continue to develop your fuelling strategy.
8. For cycling, you may wish to make a 'multi-hour bottle' and either keep concentrated or dilute to your desired consistency.

Check out our Gut-loving Gummies on page 218 for how to turn Freedom Fuel into 'sports gel chews'.

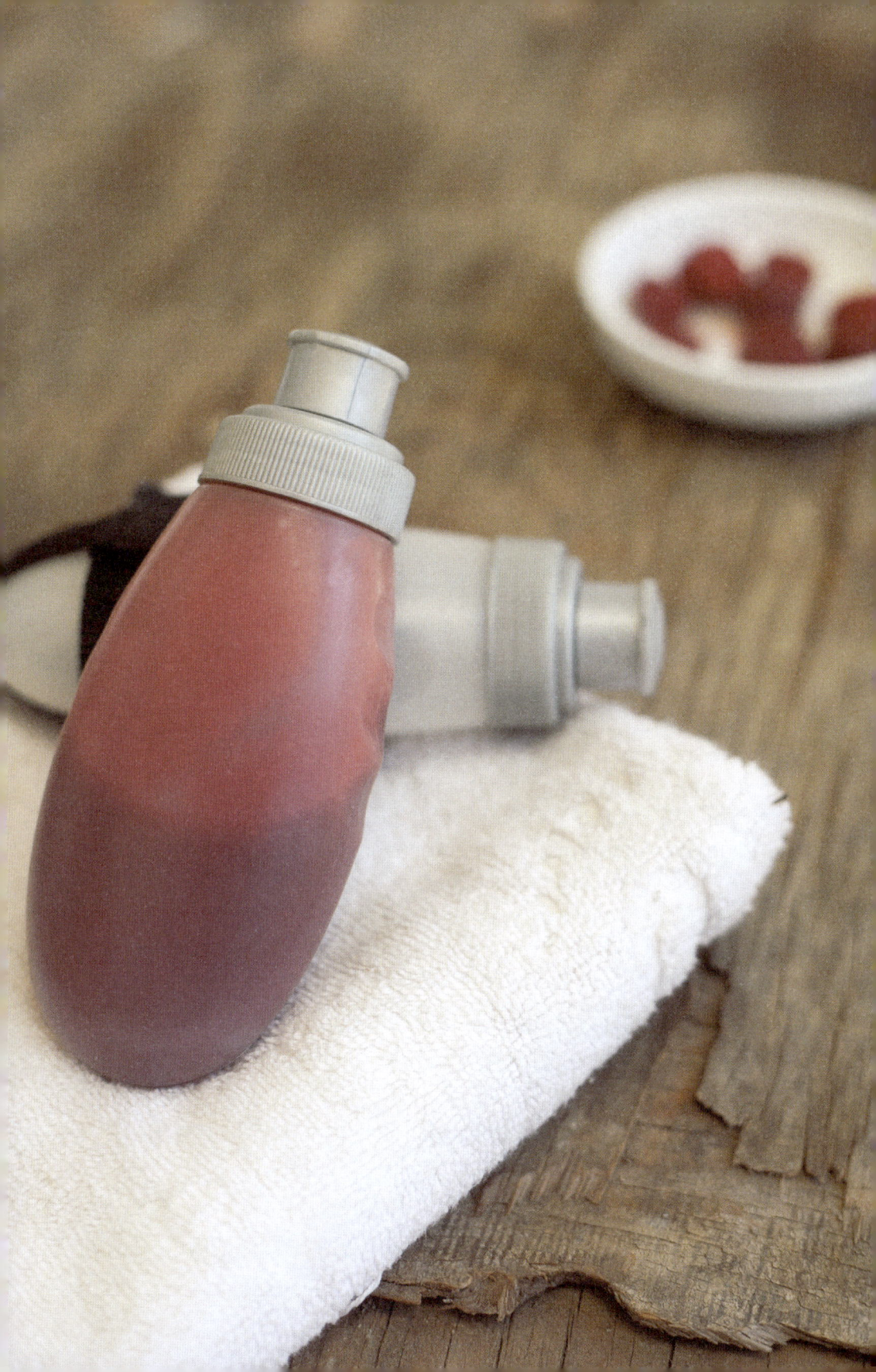

Freedom Fuel 2.0

Ingredients (Serves 1)
- 2 tablespoons cashew butter
- 4 teaspoons Pure Harvest organic rice malt syrup
- 1/4 cup blueberries
- A pinch of sea salt
- 1 teaspoon medium chain triglyceride (MCT) oil
- A dash of hot water, if required to blend

Method
1. Blend all ingredients until smooth.
2. Pour through a strainer to remove pips. Transfer carefully into a gel flask and seal well.

Note: One serve is 30g of carbohydrates, so please start to experiment with 1.0 serve/hour. For a two hour run, for example, train fasted for the first hour, then sip your 1.0 serve over the course of the second hour. Make notes of energy, digestion, performance and recovery so we can continue to develop your fuelling strategy.

Check out our Gut-loving Gummies on page 220 for how to turn Freedom Fuel into 'sports gel chews'.

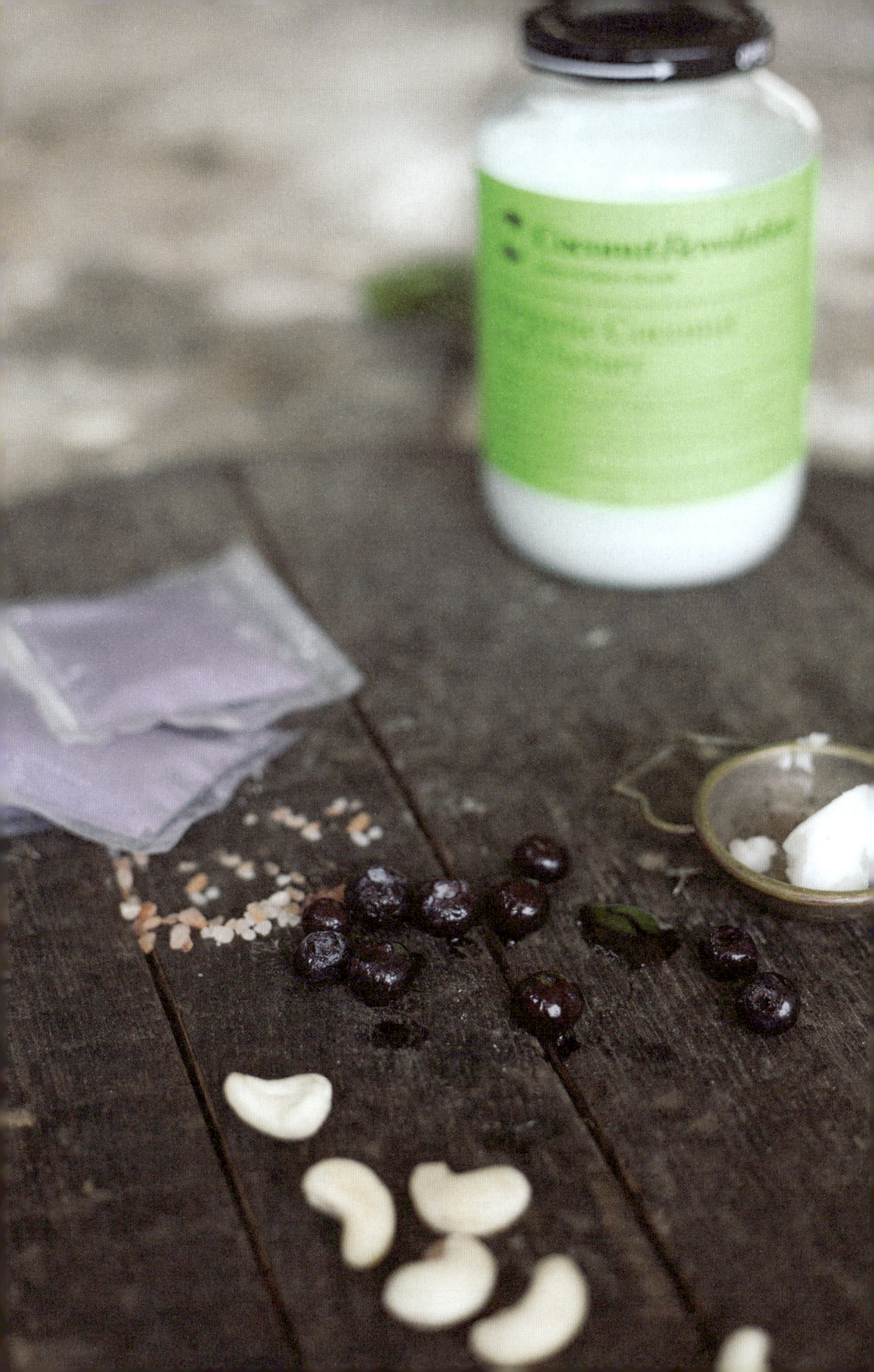

No Bake Energy Bars 1.0

Ingredients (Makes 8-10)
- 1 tablespoon cold-pressed extra virgin coconut oil
- 1 cup quinoa flakes
- 1 cup shredded unsweetened coconut
- 1/2 cup almonds, chopped
- 6-8 Medjool dates, finely chopped
- 1/4 cup cacao nibs (optional)
- 1/2 cup Pure Harvest organic rice malt syrup
- 1/4 teaspoon sea salt
- 1 teaspoon pure vanilla extract

Method
1. Preheat grill.
2. Place quinoa, coconut and almonds onto a lightly greased baking tray and toast for 5 minutes, stirring mid-way.
3. Pour toasted mix into a large bowl and stir through dates and cacao (if using).
4. In a medium saucepan, add rice malt syrup, salt and vanilla and bring to the boil (about 4-5 minutes until thick), stirring constantly. Your syrup should be thick and golden, but take care not to overcook as it will burn.
5. Pour hot syrup over dry mix and combine thoroughly.
6. Line a cookie sheet pan or cake/bread tin with greaseproof paper, or lightly coat in coconut oil.
7. Transfer mixture and press firmly until flat (grease your hands with coconut oil to prevent sticking). Feel free to sprinkle with extra coconut here.
8. Pop in the fridge to set first, then remove before slicing. Once at room temperature, cut into 8-10 bars and wrap individually in cling wrap.

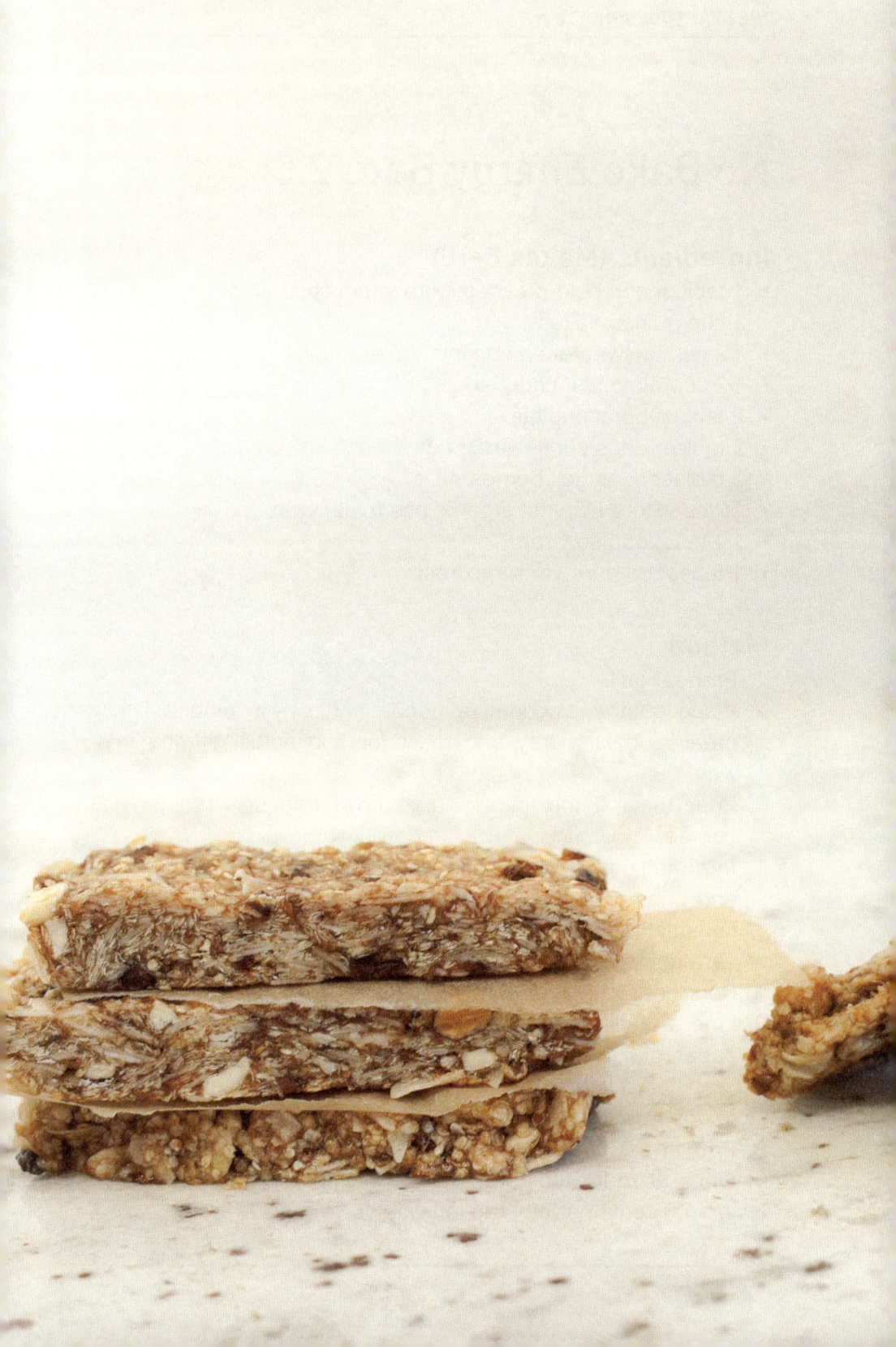

No Bake Energy Bars 2.0

Ingredients (Makes 8-10)
- 1 tablespoon cold-pressed extra virgin coconut oil
- 1 cup quinoa flakes
- 1/2 cup unsweetened coconut flakes
- 1/2 cup almonds, chopped
- 2 tablespoons pepitas
- 2 tablespoons sunflower seeds
- 2 tablespoons goji berries
- 1/2 cup Pure Harvest organic rice malt syrup
- 1/4 teaspoon sea salt
- 1 teaspoon pure vanilla extract

Method
1. Preheat grill.
2. Place quinoa, coconut, almonds and seeds onto a lightly greased baking tray and toast for 5 minutes, stirring midway.
3. Pour toasted mix into a large bowl and stir through goji berries.
4. In a medium saucepan, add rice malt syrup, salt and vanilla and bring to the boil (about 4-5 minutes until thick), stirring constantly. Your syrup should be thick and golden, but take care not to overcook as it will burn.
5. Pour hot syrup over dry mix and combine thoroughly.
6. Line a cookie sheet pan or cake/bread tin with greaseproof paper, or lightly coat in coconut oil.
7. Transfer mixture and press firmly until flat (grease your hands with coconut oil to prevent sticking).
8. Pop in the fridge to set first, then remove before slicing. Once at room temperature, cut into 8-10 bars. Store in an airtight container or wrap individually in cling wrap.

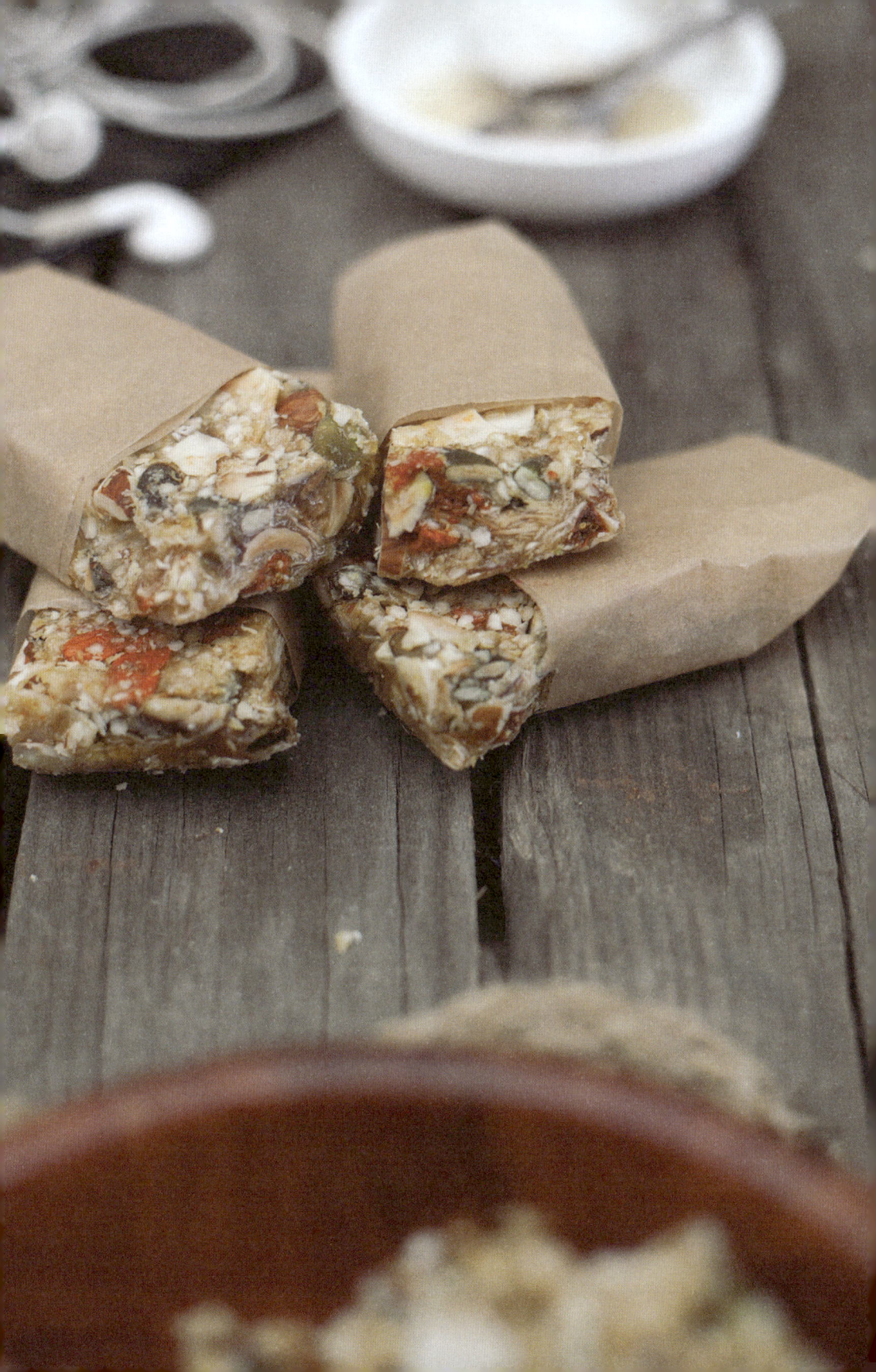

Nut Free Muesli Bars

Ingredients (Makes 8+)
- 1 cup sunflower seeds
- 1 cup pumpkin seeds
- 2 tablespoons chia seeds
- 1 cup unsweetened coconut flakes
- ¼ cup dried sour cherries
- ¼ cup cold-pressed extra virgin coconut oil
- ¼ cup + 1 tablespoon Pure Harvest organic rice malt syrup
- ¼ cup tahini
- ¼ teaspoon sea salt

Method
1. Combine seeds, coconut flakes and cherries together in a large bowl.
2. Add melted coconut oil and ¼ cup rice malt syrup and mix well.
3. In a small saucepan, heat tahini, remaining rice malt syrup and salt until well combined. Add to above mixture and combine thoroughly.
4. Transfer into a lined rectangular bread tin and compact well using the palm of your hand. The more force you apply here, the better.
5. Place in the fridge to set, before slicing into individual bars. These will keep in the fridge longer than your portion control allows.

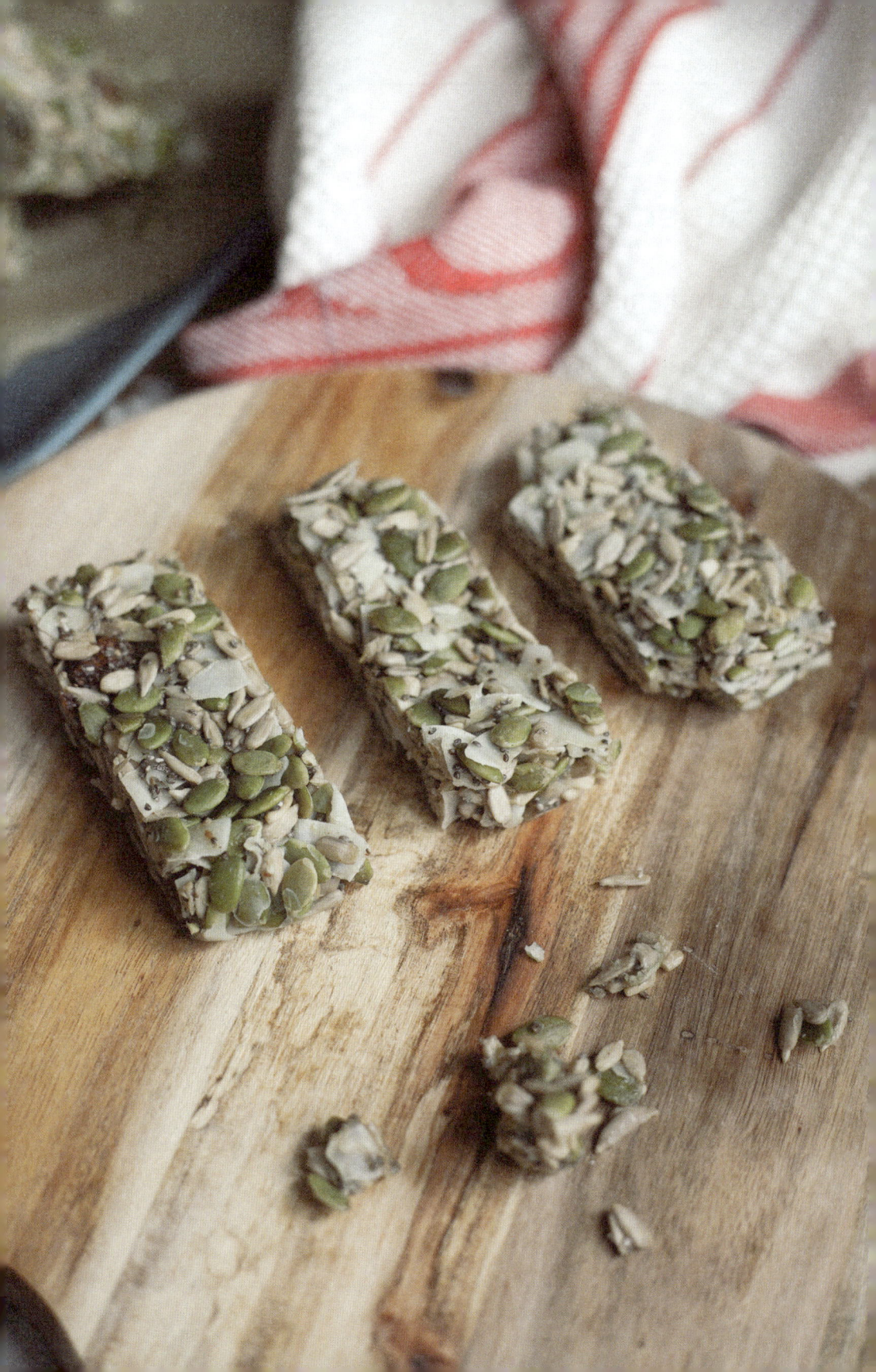

Super Easy Banana Muffins

Ingredients (Makes 12)
- 2 1/2 cups almond meal
- 1 teaspoon cinnamon
- 1 teaspoon nutmeg
- 1 teaspoon gluten free baking powder
- 4 eggs, free range
- 1/4 cup cold-pressed extra virgin coconut oil, melted
- 1/4 cup Pure Harvest organic rice malt syrup
- 1 teaspoon pure vanilla extract
- 2 bananas, mashed

Method
1. Preheat oven to 180°C.
2. In a large bowl, combine flour, cinnamon, nutmeg and baking powder.
3. In a separate bowl, beat eggs. Add to the dry mix with oil, rice malt syrup and vanilla. Stir thoroughly.
4. Add mashed banana and combine well.
5. Scoop into a greased muffin tins and bake for 35-40 minutes or until a skewer inserted comes out clean.

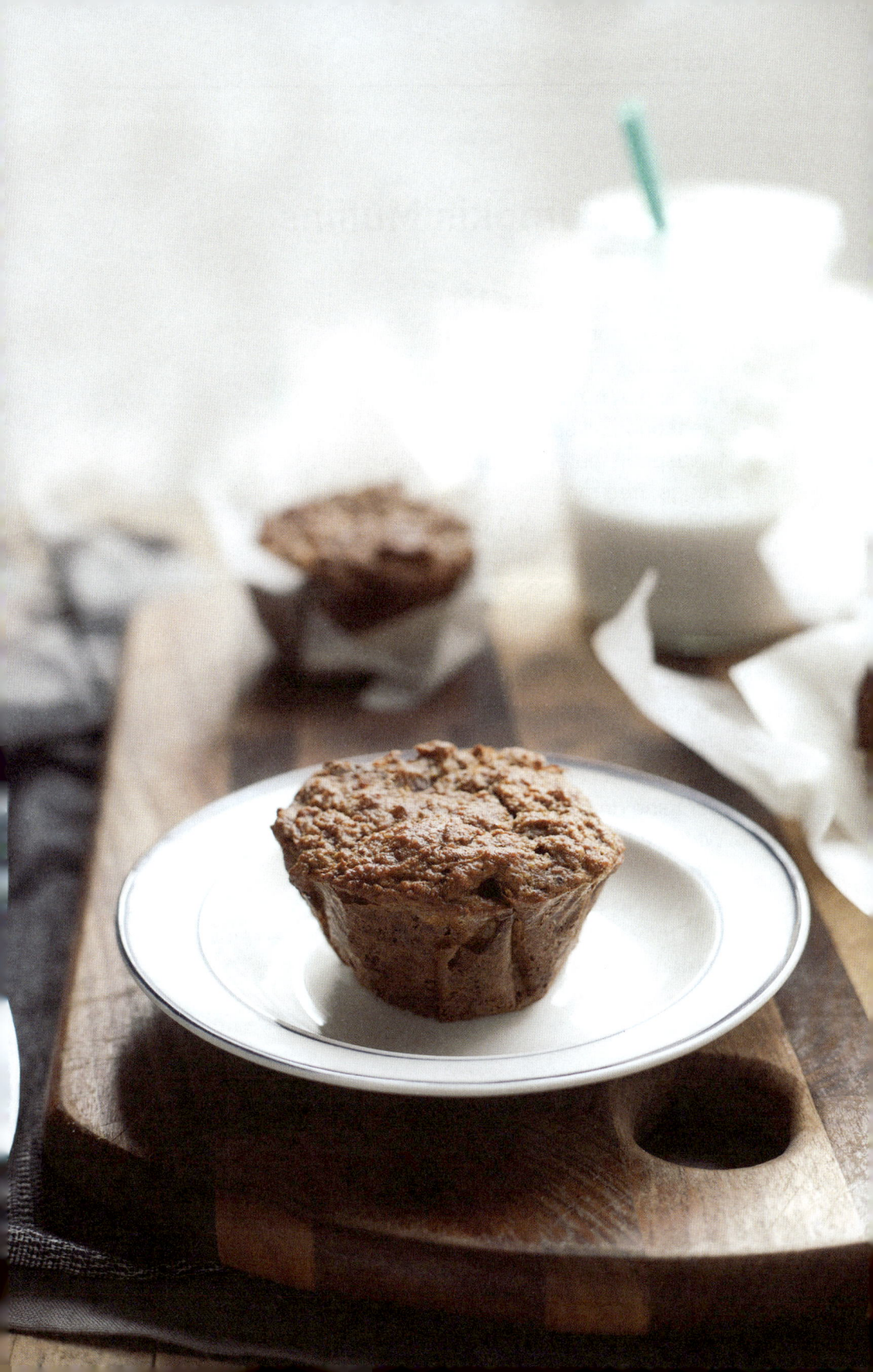

Spiced Pumpkin Muffins

Ingredients (Makes 12)
- 1/2 cup coconut flour, sifted
- 1 teaspoon cinnamon
- 1 teaspoon nutmeg
- 1 teaspoon all spice
- 1 teaspoon gluten fee baking powder
- 5 eggs, free range
- 1/2 small pumpkin or 1 cup of mashed pumpkin
- 1 teaspoon pure vanilla extract
- 1/4 cup cold-pressed extra virgin coconut oil, melted
- 1/4 cup Pure Harvest organic rice malt syrup

Method
1. Preheat oven to 180°C.
2. Remove skin and slice pumpkin into small chucks. Steam, set aside to cool and mash.
3. Combine dry ingredients together in a large bowl.
4. Whisk eggs and add with pumpkin, vanilla, oil and rice malt syrup.
5. Spoon into a greased muffin tray and bake for 30 minutes or until they pass the skewer test. Delicious served warm with a spread of organic butter.

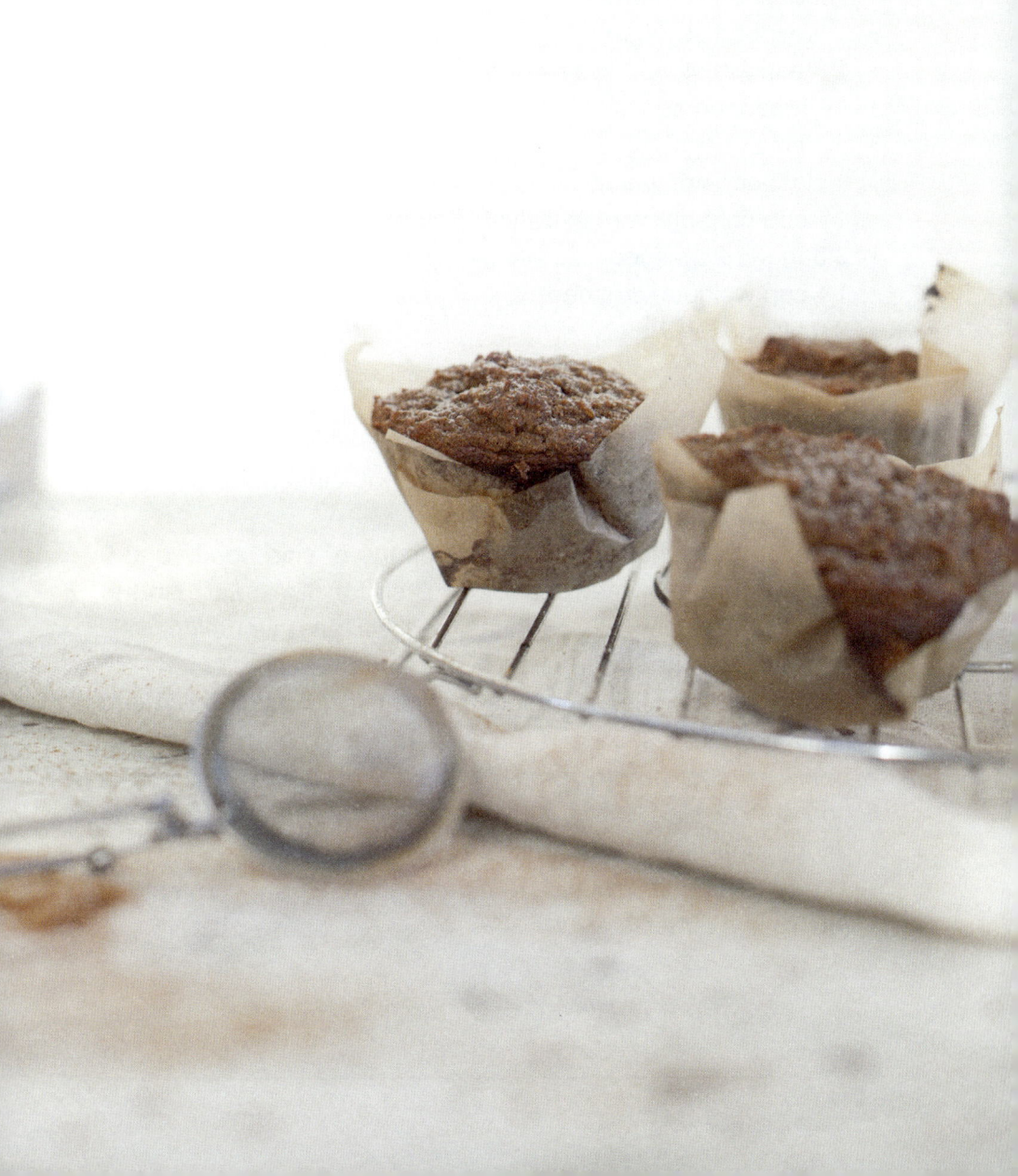

Egg Free Banana and Walnut Loaf

Ingredients
- 2 1/2 cups almond meal
- 1 teaspoon cinnamon
- 1 teaspoon psyllium
- 1 teaspoon gluten free baking powder
- 1/4 teaspoon sea salt
- 3 'chia eggs' - 3 tablespoons of chia seeds and 9 tablespoons of water
- 1/4 cup cold-pressed extra virgin coconut oil
- 3 bananas, mashed
- 1/4 cup walnuts, crushed
- 2 tablespoons water

Method
1. Preheat oven to 180°C.
2. In a large bowl, combine almond meal, cinnamon, psyllium, baking powder and salt.
3. In a separate bowl, add 3 tablespoons of chia seeds and 9 tablespoons of water and allow to sit for 5 minutes. Add to the dry mix with oil, bananas and walnuts. Combine well. Add water only if your mixture needs further combining.
4. Pour into a lightly greased loaf pan and bake for 40-45 minutes or until it passes the skewer test.
5. Allow to cool before removing from the pan. If your loaf is too soft to slice, wrap tightly in cling wrap and store in the fridge until firm. This makes 12 slices and freezes well. A great training snack and delicious served warm with a touch of organic butter.

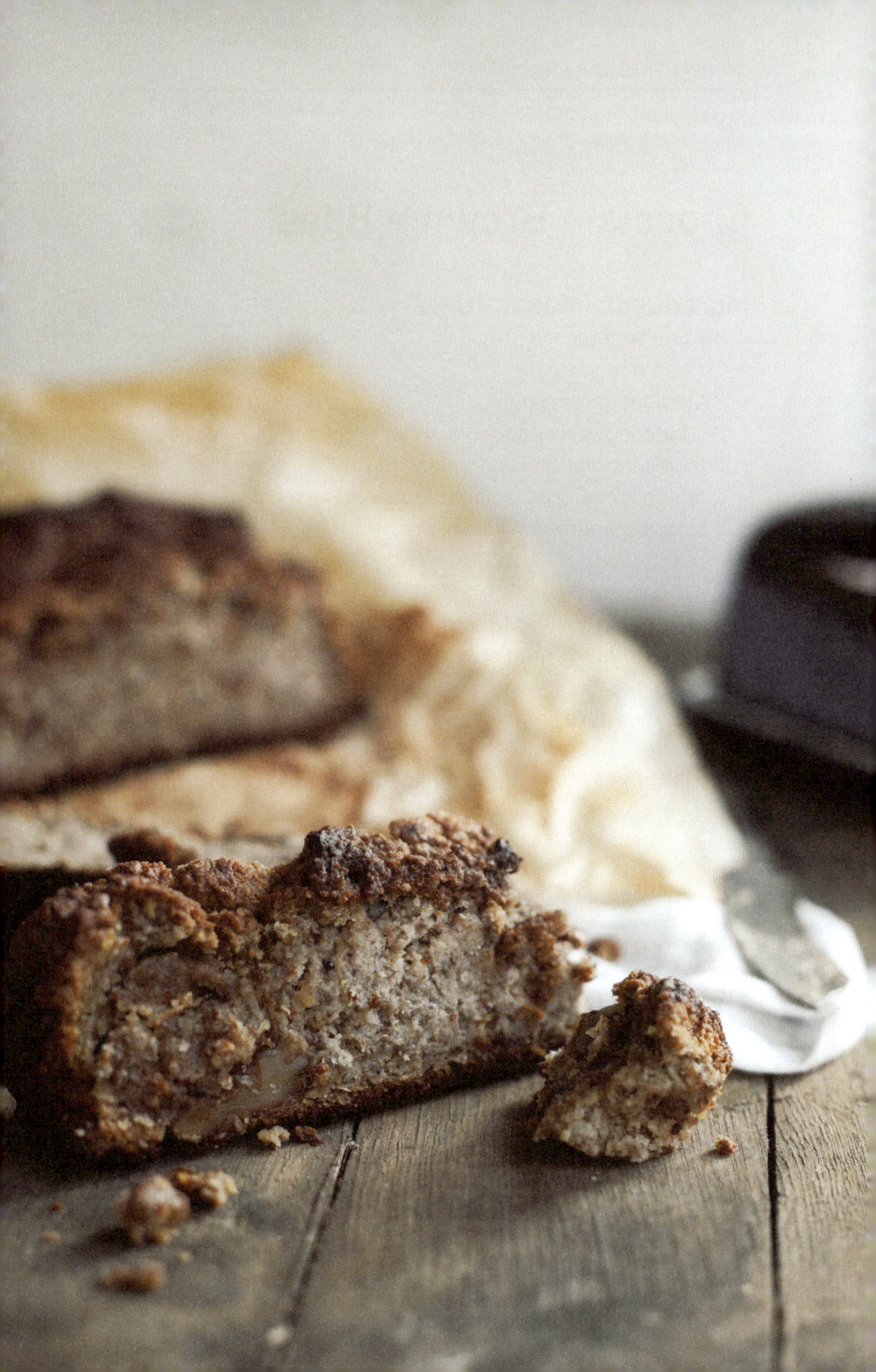

Chocolate Brownie Bites

Ingredients (Makes 10-12)
- 3/4 cup walnuts
- 1/4 cup almonds
- 8 Medjool dates, pitted
- 2 tablespoons raw cacao powder
- 2 tablespoons raw cacao nibs
- 2 tablespoons unsweetened coconut flakes
- 1 teaspoon pure vanilla extract

Method
1. Blend nuts together to form fine nut flour.
2. Add all other ingredients and blend until a crumbly mixture forms.
3. Empty mixture into a bowl and roll palm size scoops into balls.
4. Chill in the fridge before serving and freeze prior to training.

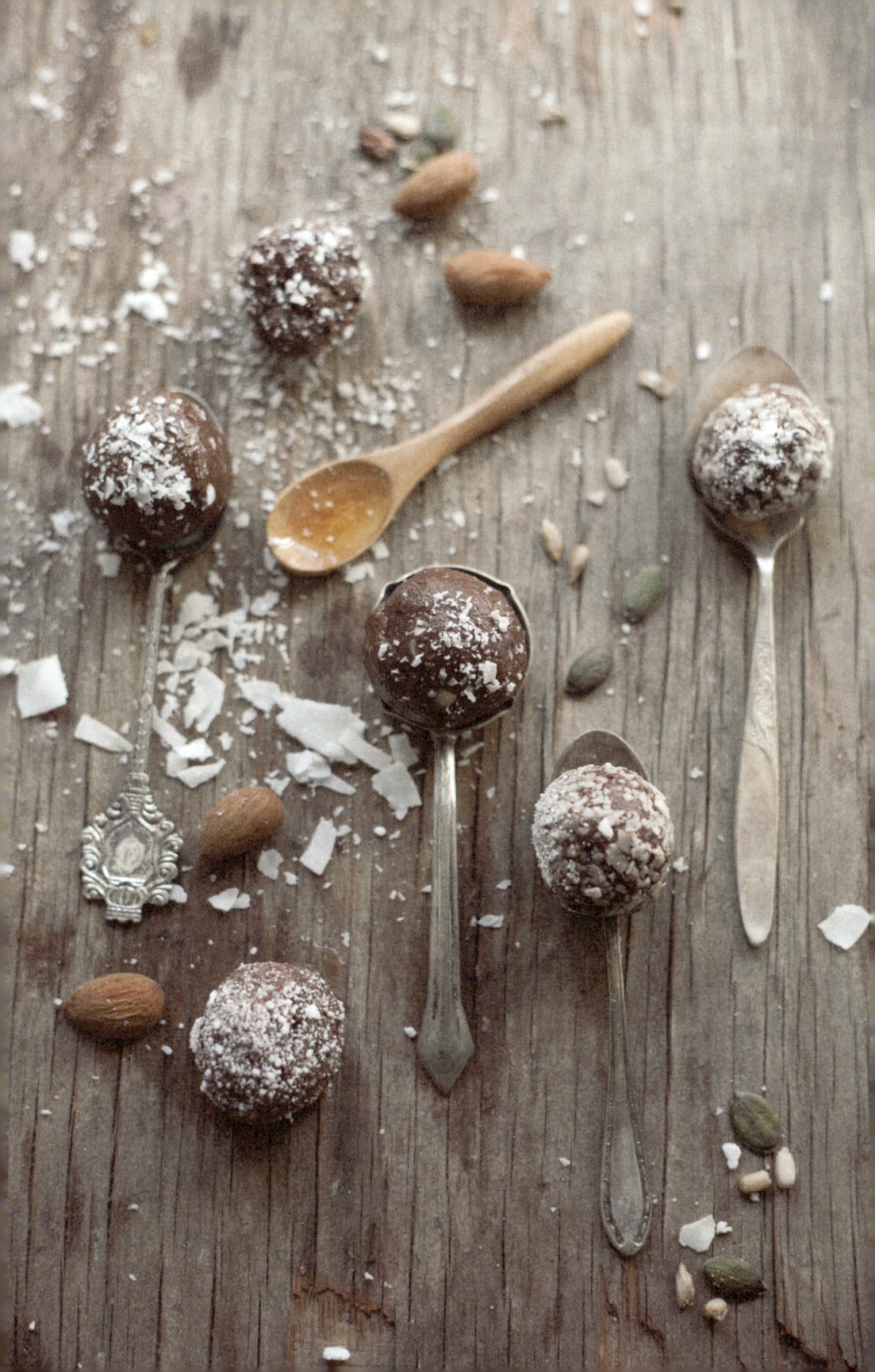

Raw Cashew and Chia Protein Bites

Ingredients (Makes 8-10)
- 250g cashews
- 1 scoop of quality protein powder, such as Bare Blends
- 2 tablespoons cacao powder
- 1 - 1 1/2 tablespoons Natvia, depending on desired sweetness
- 1 tablespoon cinnamon
- 1/4 cup cold-pressed extra virgin coconut oil
- 1 tablespoon chia seeds
- 1/4 cup water

Method
1. Blend the nuts, protein powder, cacao, Natvia and cinnamon and add to a large bowl.
2. Add the melted coconut oil and stir well.
3. Add the chia seeds and water after soaking for 10 minutes.
4. Use an ice cream scoop or spoon and form balls that sit nicely in the palm of your hand. To prevent sticking, add a touch of oil to your hands prior to doing so. Makes 8-10.

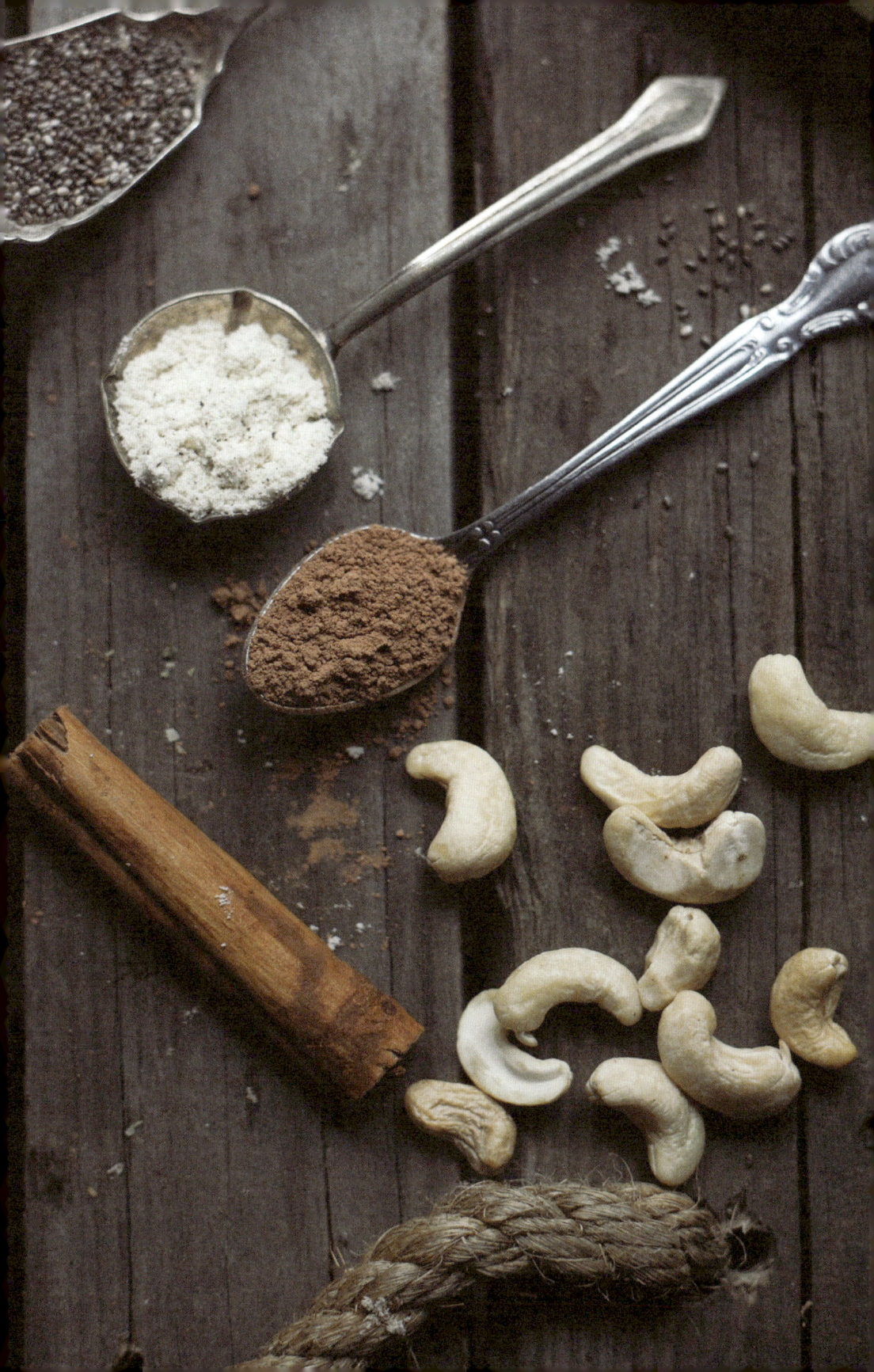

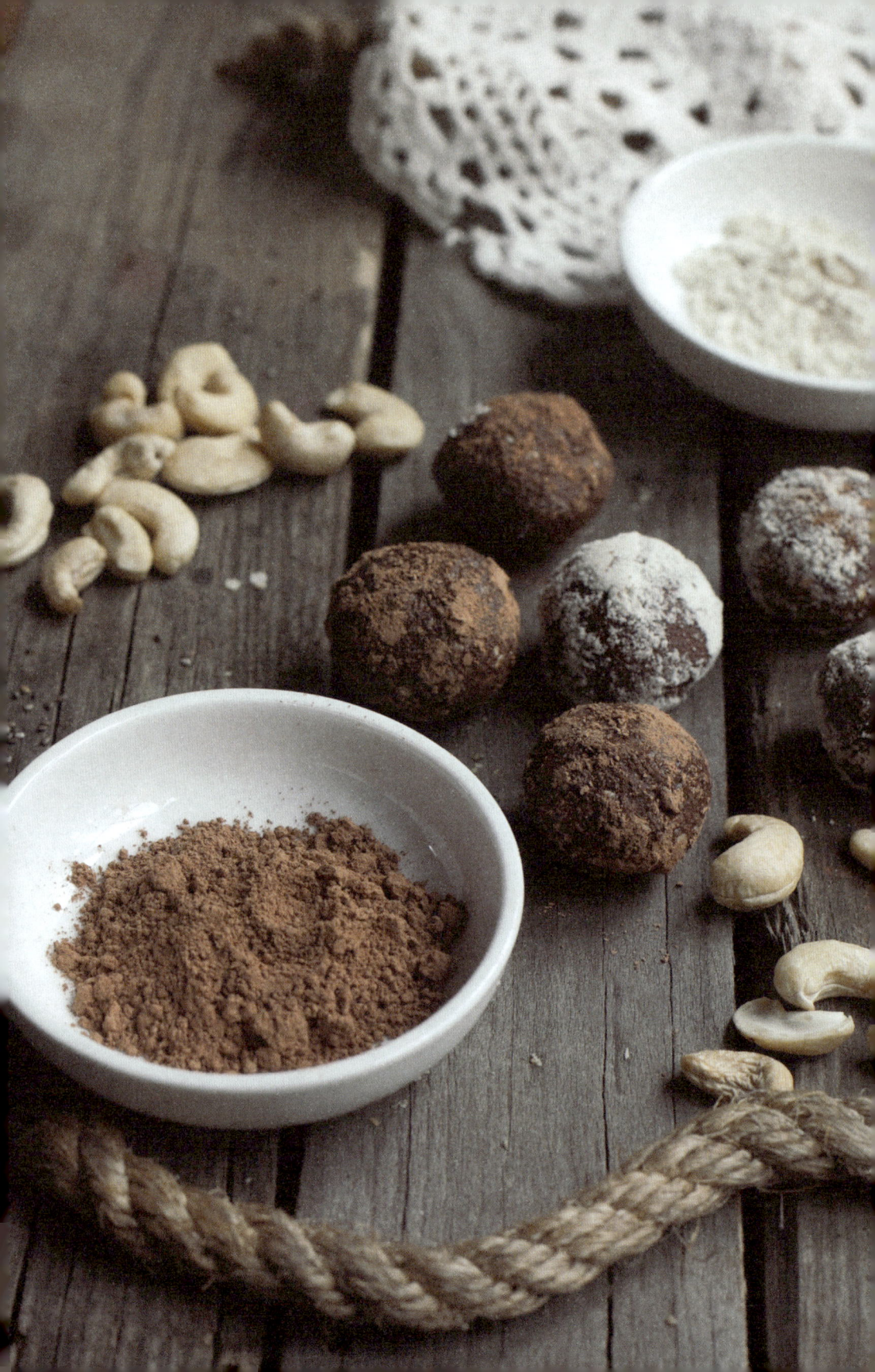

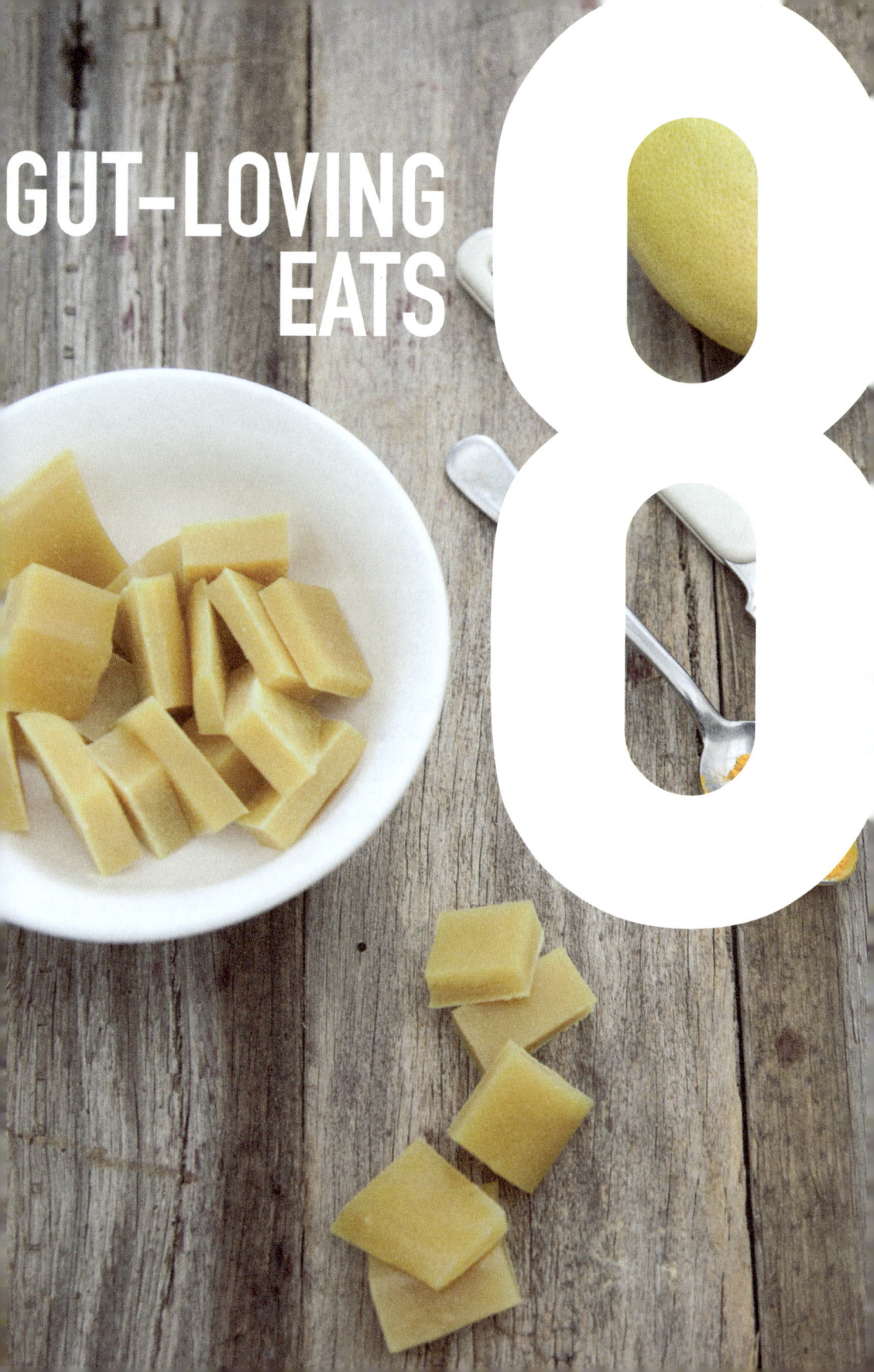

GUT-LOVING EATS

8

Super Easy Bone Broth

Ingredients
- 0.5kg beef bones or oxtail or 1 chicken carcass (always free-range and grass-fed)
- Enough water to completely cover bones
- 2 tablespoons apple cider vinegar (ACV) (this helps to extract the calcium)
- A pinch of sea salt

Method
1. In a large pot or slow cooker, combine all ingredients.
2. Bring to the boil on the stove before simmering for 48-72 hours.
3. Allow to cool before straining and retain only the liquid yield. There will be fat to skim off and potentially leftover bone, depending on which time frame you chose. (Please note: if you use chicken, most of the bones should have dissolved. Expect to have bones left if you use beef or oxtail, which you can re-use for your next batch).
4. Serve warm or reheated on the stove and aim to drink one small cup per day.

Bone broth tips and tricks
- *Keep what you will use in the next few days in a glass container in the fridge.*
- *Freeze the rest into single serves to drink with a meal or to use as stock for soups, stews and any recipe requiring stock. Your bone broth will last a few months in the freezer. A great space saving tip is to freeze in silicon muffin trays before transferring into zip lock bags.*
- *Freeze in ice cube trays or muffins trays and defrost a few at a time as required.*
- *After 24 hours of cooking time, add vegetables such as garlic, onion, carrots, celery and zucchini for flavour and variety.*

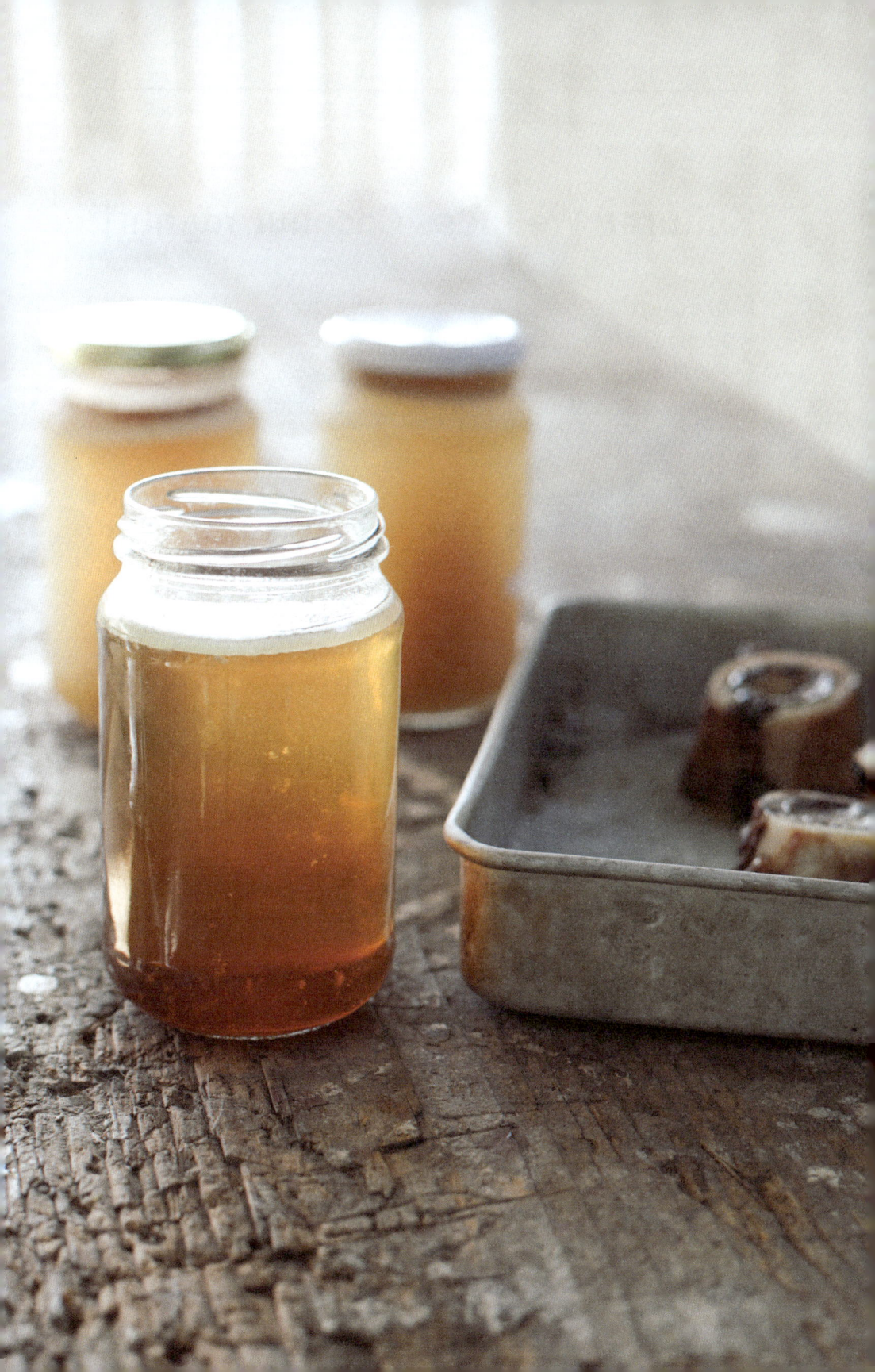

Kultured Wellness Coconut Yoghurt

Ingredients
- 1600ml of Ayam coconut cream (4 x 400ml cans)
- 1 Kultured Wellness Yoghurt Starter (www.thenaturalnutritionist.com.au/kultured-wellness/)

Method
1. Place the ingredients into a food processor or blender and blend on the lowest speed until smooth and combined. Alternatively, you may just stir ingredients together in a large ceramic or glass bowl with a wooden spoon. Avoid metal or plasticware for this recipe, the cultures corode the metal, whilst toxins from the plastic may leach into your food.
2. Transfer to a large glass container, leaving ample amount of room at the top of the jar, as the yoghurt may expand during the ferment.
3. Secure the lid and leave the mixture to ferment for 8-12 hours. Taste after 8 hours. The yoghurt should be tangy and rid any detectable sweetness, if it is ready, transfer to the fridge, if it's still sweet, leave for the rest of the fermenting time before transferring to the fridge.
4. Keep one cup from this batch to start the next batch. You may repeat this method 5 times before you will need to replenish your starter supply from Kultured Wellness.

Start by consuming a quarter of a cup per day and work your way up to one cup per day over a four week period. It's great added to smoothies or served with fresh berries.

Kultured Wellness Coconut Kefir

Ingredients
- 1 Kultured Wellness Kefir starter (www.thenaturalnutritionist.com.au/kultured-wellness/)
- Coconut water (about 1.7L)

Method
1. Place both ingredients in a 2L glass jar, leaving some space between the liquid and the top of the jar, in case the liquid fizzes and expands during the ferment.
2. Stir liquid with a wooden spoon and leave on the bench to ferment for 24-48 hours, tasting after 24 hours. The kefir should be tangy with no detectable coconut sweetness. In warmer weather it will ferment in 24 hours and for cooler climates 48 hours is needed for all the sugar to be eaten up by the beneficial bacteria.
3. Once the kefir is ready, use 1 cup to start your next batch and transfer the rest to the fridge. You can make 10L of coconut water from your initial starter (saving 1 cup per 2L batch), before replenishing your starter supply from Kultured Wellness.

Start by consuming a quarter of a cup per day and work your way up to one cup per day over a four week period. Simply drink with a meal or use post-training as a great way to rehydrate.

Gut-loving Gummies - Raspberry

Ingredients
- 1/3 cup water
- 3 1/2 tablespoons gelatin powder
- 2 teaspoons Pure Harvest organic rice malt syrup
- 1 teaspoon cold-pressed extra virgin coconut oil
- 1/4 cup frozen raspberries
- The juice of 1/4 lemon
- A pinch of sea salt

Method
1. Dissolve the gelatin in 1/3 cup of cold water and let it sit for 5 minutes to become gel-like. It will firm immediately so stir quickly and leave it until a rubber ball-like consistency forms.
2. Heat the rice malt syrup, coconut oil, raspberries, lemon juice and salt in a saucepan until the fruit has softened. Puree using a stick blender and stir in the gelatin. Remove from heat.
3. Pour into a 10 x 15 cm glass or plastic container. Refrigerate for 1 hour then cut into squares. Store in the fridge for up to 5-7 days and consume 3-4 per day.

This recipe doubles as one serve of Freedom Fuel Chews. Consume as per guidelines on page 192, for example 1.5-2.0 serves/hour.

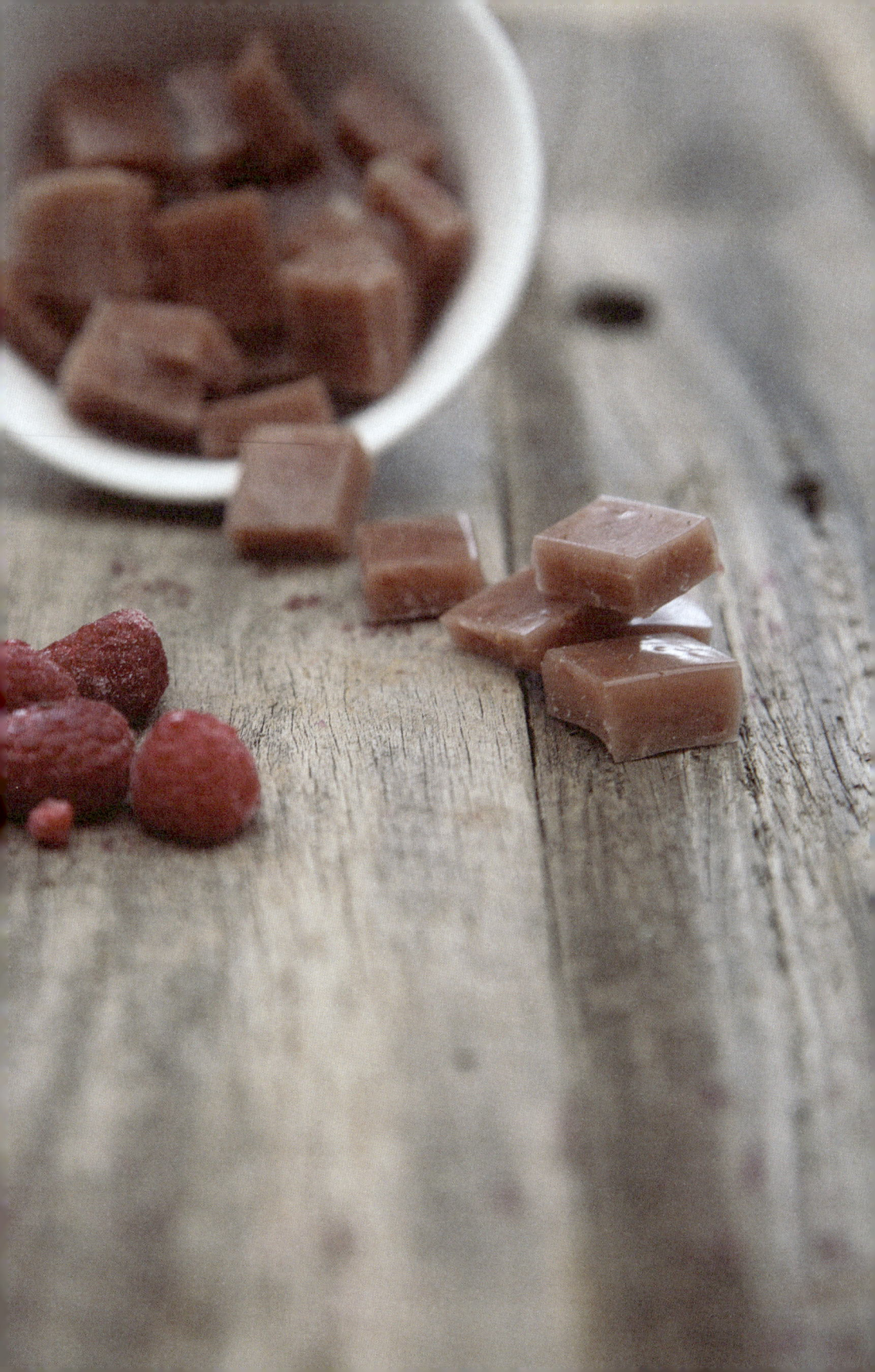

Gut-loving Gummies - Blueberry

Ingredients
- 1/3 cup water
- 3 1/2 tablespoons gelatin powder
- 2 teaspoons Pure Harvest organic rice malt syrup
- 1 teaspoon cold-pressed extra virgin coconut oil
- 1/4 cup frozen blueberries
- The juice of 1/4 lemon
- A pinch of sea salt

Method
1. Dissolve the gelatin in 1/3 cup of cold water and let it sit for 5 minutes to become gel-like. It will firm immediately so stir quickly and leave it until a rubber ball-like consistency forms.
2. Heat the rice malt syrup, coconut oil, blueberries, lemon juice and salt in a saucepan until the fruit has softened. Puree using a stick blender and stir in the gelatin. Remove from heat.
3. Pour into a 10 x 15 cm glass or plastic container. Refrigerate for 1 hour then cut into squares. Store in the fridge for up to 5-7 days and consume 3-4 per day.

This recipe doubles as one serve of Freedom Fuel Chews. Consume as per guidelines on page 194, for example 1.5 serves/hour.

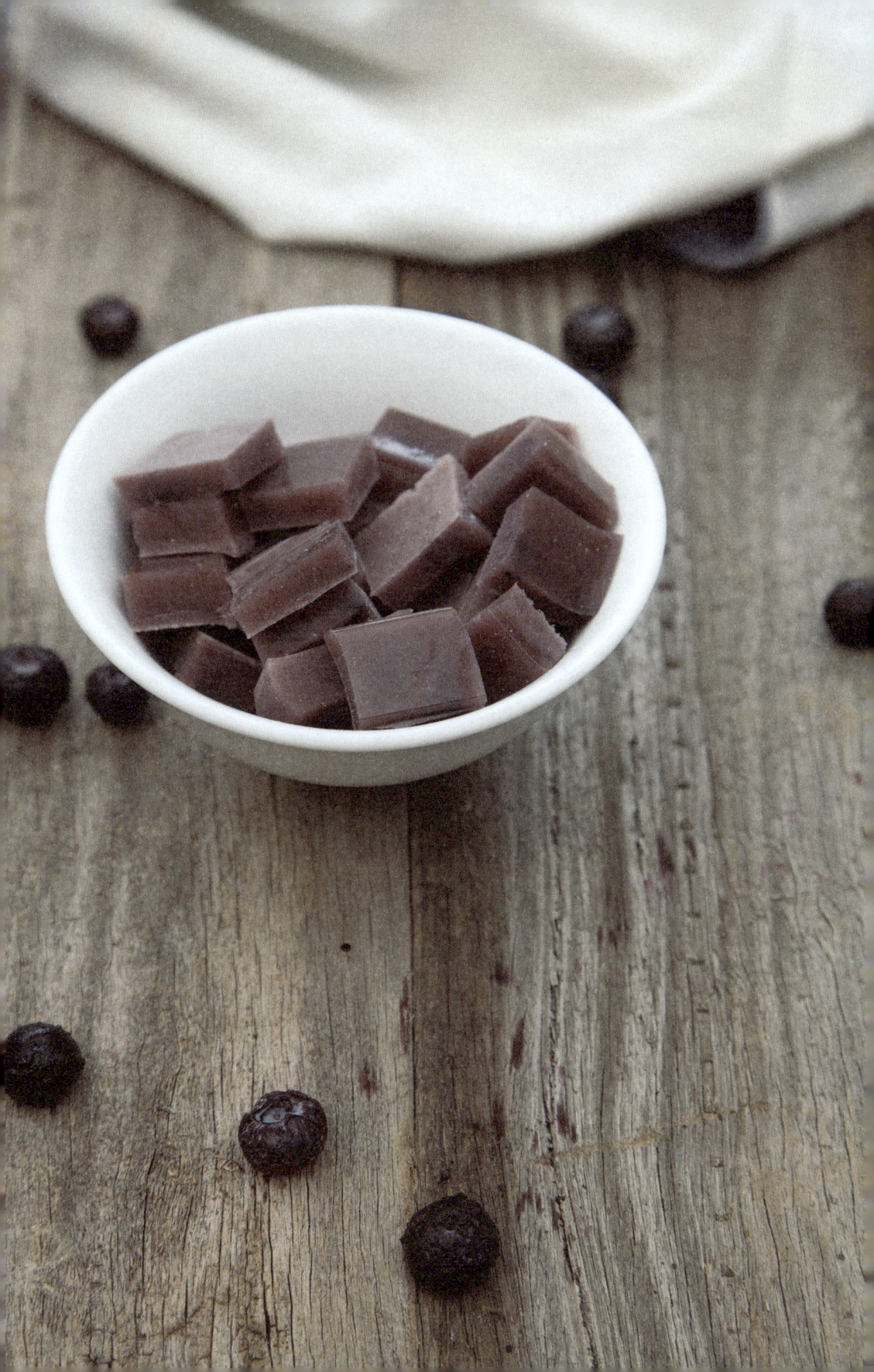

Gut-loving Gummies - Lemon

Ingredients
- 1/3 cup water
- 3 1/2 tablespoons gelatin powder
- 2 teaspoons Pure Harvest organic rice malt syrup
- 1 teaspoon cold-pressed extra virgin coconut oil
- 1/4 teaspoon turmeric
- The juice of 1/2 lemon
- A pinch of sea salt

Method
1. Dissolve the gelatin in 1/3 cup of cold water and let it sit for 5 minutes to become gel-like. It will firm immediately so stir quickly and leave it until a rubber ball-like consistency forms.
2. Heat the rice malt syrup, coconut oil, turmeric, lemon juice and salt in a saucepan. Stir in the gelatin and remove from heat.
3. Pour into a 10 x 15 cm glass or plastic container. Refrigerate for 1 hour then cut into squares. Store in the fridge for up to 5-7 days and consume 3-4 per day.

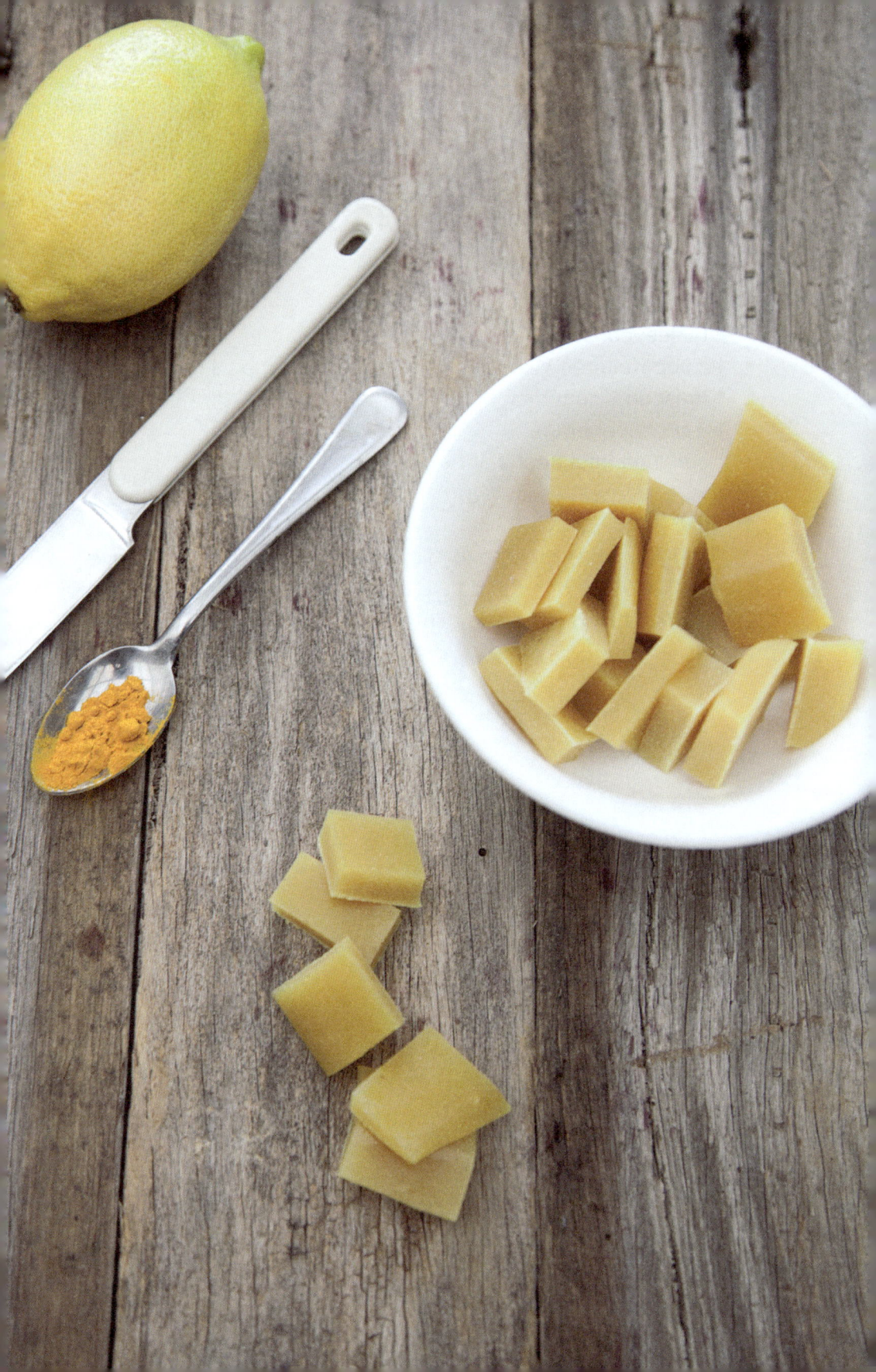

Fermented Chia Pudding

Ingredients (Serves 1)
- 2 tablespoons chia seeds
- 1/2 cup Kultured Wellness Coconut Kefir (page 217)
- 1 teaspoon cinnamon
- 1/2 cup blueberries
- 1 small handful fresh mint

Method
1. Combine chia, kefir and cinnamon in and jar and leave overnight (8-12 hours) on the bench top to ferment.
2. Top with blueberries and mint to serve.

Do you need personalised support with your real food journey?

One-on-one consultations are available in the south-eastern suburbs of Melbourne. Skype and phone consultations are also available - we have clients Australia-wide and overseas.

If you are ready to get started with your personalised nutrition straight away, please book your Initial Consultation online at bit.ly/tnnonline. Please use the promotion code **JERF** upon booking, as we are happy to offer you 10% off all of our services for investing in your health with this book.

If you would like to discuss your needs and/or have us help you select from our program options, please contact us at www.thenaturalnutritionist.com.au/contact/

Find out more about us www.thenaturalnutritionist.com.au/about

Yours in health,

Steph and the team at The Natural Nutritionist.

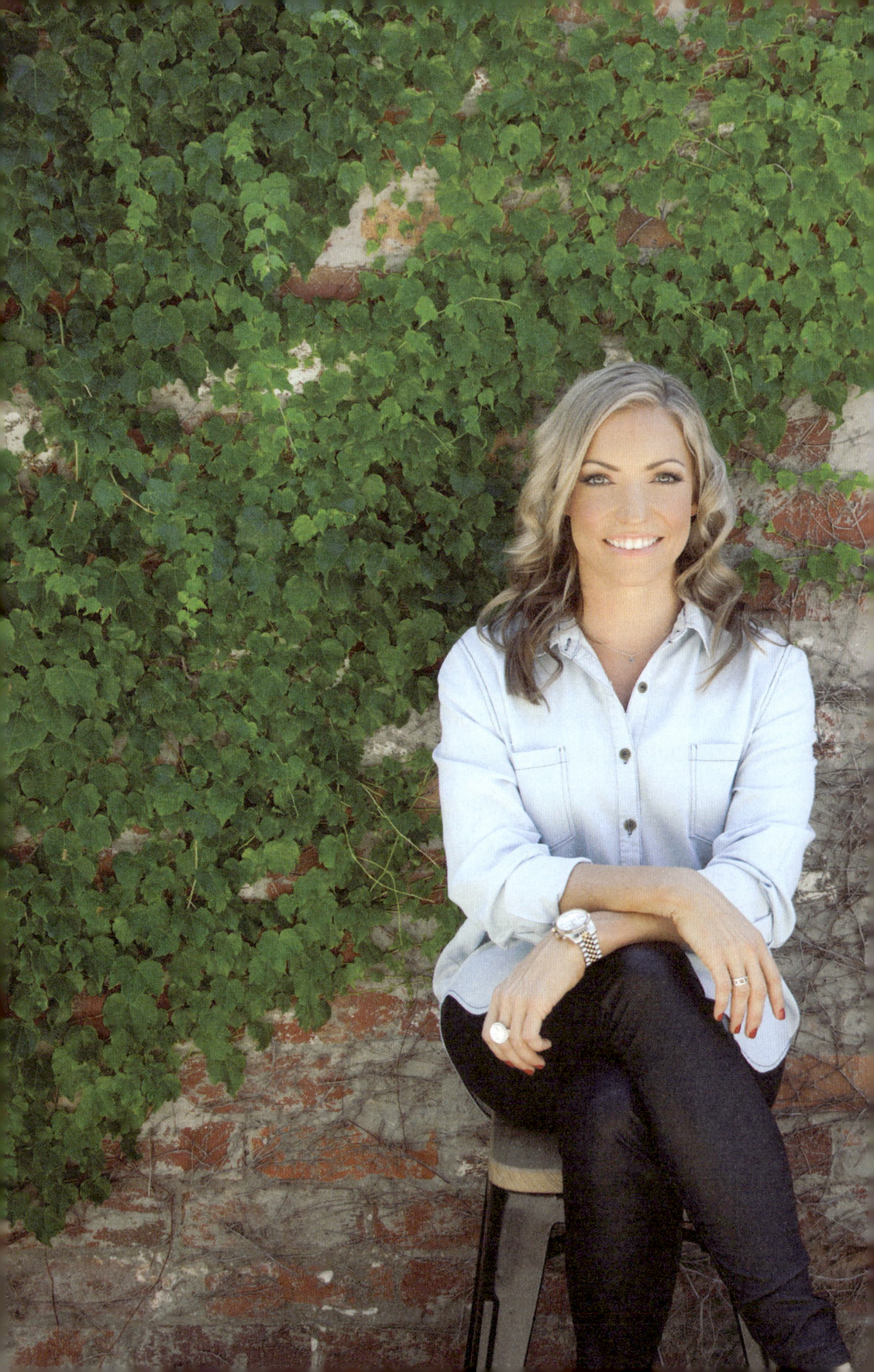

Thank You

Dr Phil Maffetone, thank you for being the pioneer, for without your work I may have never stumbled across my purpose in life.

Tim Noakes, Bob Seebohar, Jeff Volek and Stephen Phinney - my additional industry idols, thank you for starting and continuing the conversation, your research, and for putting up a fight when conventionalism strikes.

My sister Angela, for your advice, support, belief and love.

Ian, for inspiring me to play big.

My photographer Sarah Craven, who takes the creative rein and makes my life much easier and this book, much better looking.

My athletes. For being my guiding lights, Guinea pigs and biggest supporters. It's a pleasure to guide you through your real food journey.

You. Thank you for your support in purchasing this book and continuing to spread The Real Food Athlete love. It's a dream come true.

© The Natural Nutritionist 2016